divine indulgences

divine indulgences

rose reisman's sensational light desserts

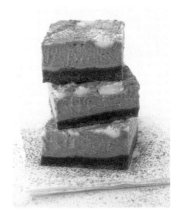

PENGUIN
CANADA

PENGUIN CANADA

Published by the Penguin Group

Penguin Group (Canada), 10 Alcorn Avenue, Toronto, Ontario, Canada M4V 3B2
    (a division of Pearson Penguin Canada Inc.)

Penguin Group (USA) Inc., 375 Hudson Street, New York, New York 10014, U.S.A.
Penguin Books Ltd, 80 Strand, London WC2R 0RL, England
Penguin Ireland, 25 St Stephen's Green, Dublin 2, Ireland (a division of Penguin Books Ltd)
Penguin Group (Australia), 250 Camberwell Road, Camberwell, Victoria 3124, Australia
    (a division of Pearson Australia Group Pty Ltd)
Penguin Books India Pvt Ltd, 11 Community Centre, Panchsheel Park, New Delhi – 110 017, India
Penguin Group (NZ), Cnr Airborne and Rosedale Roads, Albany, Auckland, New Zealand
    (a division of Pearson New Zealand Ltd)
Penguin Books (South Africa) (Pty) Ltd, 24 Sturdee Avenue, Rosebank, Johannesburg 2196, South Africa

Penguin Books Ltd, Registered Offices: 80 Strand, London WC2R 0RL, England

First published by Prentice Hall Canada, a division of Pearson Penguin Canada Inc., 2001
Published in Penguin Canada paperback by Penguin Group (Canada), a division of
    Pearson Penguin Canada Inc., 2003

(KR) 10 9 8 7 6 5 4 3 2

Manufactured in Canada.

LIBRARY AND ARCHIVES CANADA CATALOGUING IN PUBLICATION

Reisman, Rose, 1953–
    Divine indulgences : Rose Reisman's sensational light desserts.

Includes index.

1. Desserts. 2. Low-fat diet—Recipes. I. Title.

TX773.R452 2003   641.8'6   C2003-902447-4

Visit the Penguin Group (Canada) website at **www.penguin.ca**

I have a joy and zest for life.
I owe this spirit to the most important people in my life:

My husband, Sam, with whom I'm about to celebrate our 25th wedding anniversary (I can't believe we made it). He truly is the "light" of my life and has always encouraged me to do what I want, whether he agreed with me or not. I love him to pieces.

My daughter Natalie: the intense, disciplined, capable and wonderful oldest child.

My son David: the cool, sensitive, balanced and easygoing oldest son.

My daughter Laura: a free spirit, and the emotional and spiritual youngest daughter.

My baby Adam: a wonderfully whimsical, imaginative son and the true "child" in my family.

And I can't forget my German shepherds, Aspen and Meiko, who give me my tranquility each day as we trek through the woods.

This is all that matters.

contents

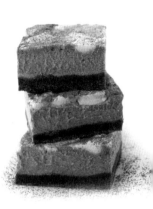

acknowledgments

To all the "divine" people who made this book as "delicious" as it could be.

Thanks to the entire crew at Pearson PTR Canada, including Nicole de Montbrun, Andrea Crozier and Ed Carson, for all their care and confidence in this book, and in me. And a big thanks to Tracy Bordian, who kept this book to an incredibly tight and high-pressure schedule with ease. That's impressive!

Thanks to Martin Litkowski and Jennifer Matyczak, who have been responsible for making me visible across the country.

Thanks to an amazing editor, Madeline Koch, for forcing me—late at night—to get her my changes. She was great to work with.

As always, to my assistant Lesleigh Landry, for sampling hundreds of desserts. She not only assisted in the testing but also helped turn my illegible handwriting into readable script. Thanks, also, for assistance in the nutritional analyses.

Thanks to the assistants in my home, Lily Lim and Ruby Reveche, who always made sure there were ample ingredients and utensils.

Thanks to all those "great" friends, especially Susan Gordin and Kathy Kacer, who stopped by each night to pick up extra dessert for their family and friends. And who gave me honest criticism for each dessert. Sometimes too honest!

foreword

At last! Here's the book I've always wanted to write: one devoted exclusively to desserts.

And not just any desserts—these are desserts you can *really* enjoy, because not only are they wonderfully satisfying, they're also amazingly low in fat and calories.

All of the pleasure, none of the guilt. Now *that's* a divine indulgence.

The origins of this book go back to the 1980s, when I made my first attempt at writing a cookbook. Would-be authors are always told to "write what you know," which made my choice of subjects easy: desserts, of course. So I put together a collection of my favourite dessert recipes and, chocolate- and butter-stained manuscript in hand, made the rounds to all the major book publishers.

My efforts were not exactly a resounding success. The publishing people were very nice about it, but made it clear that they weren't interested in a dessert book from an unknown author. At the time, I was devastated. But in retrospect, it was probably the best thing that could have happened.

Those original recipes were everything I thought a dessert should be: sinfully rich, with loads of butter, cream, eggs and chocolate. And they *were* delicious. But not long after my first attempts to get published, a visit to the doctor—and a report that my cholesterol levels were off the scale—forced me to look at food in an entirely different way. From that came my "conversion" to light cooking and my first really big success as a cookbook author.

Today, with nine cookbooks behind me, totaling more than 750,000 copies, I'm finally able to write my dessert book. And it's been worth the wait. Over the years, I've had the opportunity to develop and refine my light cooking techniques to create desserts that are healthy yet unbelievably satisfying. In fact, I've found that many of them actually taste *better* without all the extra fat.

But don't take my word for it. Just sample any of the recipes (more than 200 of them) in this book, including cheesecakes, coffee cakes, layer cakes, cobblers, pies, tarts, cookies, brownies, soufflés, puddings and sauces, as well as exotic desserts that will impress any crowd. Some of my personal favourites include Banana Chocolate Fudge Layer Cake, Date Oatmeal Coffee Cake, Pecan Cream Cheese Pie, and Chocolate Sour Cream Cheesecake Squares.

Every recipe in this book has been tested a minimum of four times. Only those that meet my dessert-lover's standards for flavour, moistness, texture and appearance have been included. (No "pretty good for low-fat" desserts here.) I've also provided a comprehensive nutritional analysis for each recipe (if only because you might not otherwise believe it's lower in fat), as well as a special section on soy-based desserts for people who can't eat dairy foods.

One of the most popular classes at my cooking school (which opened in September 2000) is "Desserts to Die For." At the end of each session, as we're sampling the recipes, my students always ask me how low-fat desserts can taste so good. The secret, as you'll discover in this book, is to use all those wonderful higher-fat ingredients you love, but in smaller quantities. Eating well—and living well—is really just a question of finding the right balance.

So get out your baking pans and discover just how easy it is to make the most divinely light desserts you've ever tasted.

Enjoy!

Rose

divine indulgences

the divine light dessert: an introduction

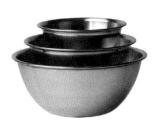

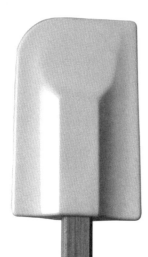

general techniques for lowering the fat in desserts

1. First, you must know where the fat is coming from. The main sources are butter, margarine, oil, eggs, sour cream, whipping cream, chocolate, nuts, and cream cheese.

2. Do not try to eliminate the fat. You are trying to find sources so you can reduce the amount.

3. You can successfully reduce approximately 50% to 75% of the fat in a traditional recipe using substitutions. Keep at least 25% of the fat for flavour and texture.

4. Fat can be substituted with low-fat yogurt, low-fat sour cream, buttermilk, low-fat evaporated milk, puréed fruits such as bananas or pineapple, or cooked puréed fruits such as dried dates, prunes, apricots, applesauce, and figs.

5. A combination of low-fat ricotta or cottage cheese and a small amount of light cream cheese can replace high-fat cream cheese.

6. For each whole egg you can use 2 egg whites. I like to keep some of the egg yolks in a recipe for flavour and texture. Too many egg whites will make a cake tough and rubbery.

7. Cocoa can replace the chocolate in a recipe. Cocoa is much lower in fat and calories than chocolate. I often use a small amount of chocolate to highlight the chocolate taste in a recipe.

8. Instead of a buttery piecrust, I use cookie crumb crusts held together mostly with water and just a small amount of fat.

9. To make delicious crunchy toppings, I use quick-cooking oats or a crunchy cereal like Grape-Nuts to replace the nuts traditionally used.

10. Instead of whipping cream for mousses, I use beaten egg whites in combination with a ricotta base, which gives wonderful volume and texture without excess calories and fat. A small amount of gelatin helps to hold the texture of the dessert.

11. Using low-fat evaporated milk or low-fat condensed milk instead of heavy cream gives the dessert a creamy, rich consistency.

12. The proper ingredients make the success of any dessert. Always check the freshness of your ingredients before storing them. If they are stale or old, they won't function properly in your dessert and may in fact destroy it.

dry ingredients
flour

The flour used in most of my recipes is all-purpose flour. This flour is often a blend of 80% plain flour and 20% cake flour. It is excellent for all cakes and cookies except for those that specify cake flour, which is milled from soft wheat and has a lower gluten level, and is specifically designed to produce a tender grain in cakes. You can make your own cake flour from all-purpose flour by substituting 2 tbsp cornstarch for 2 tbsp flour in every cup. To substitute cake flour for all-purpose flour, use 1 cup plus 2 tbsp cake flour for every cup of all-purpose flour.

Unbleached flour is more nutritious because some of the wheat bran is retained during the milling and refining process. It tends to be a little heavier than bleached flour and is not desirable for delicate cakes.

Whole-wheat flour is not milled as finely as white flour and contains much of the bran and wheat germ, making it darker, coarser, and more nutritious. If you're going to substitute this flour for white flour, use up to 50% of whole-wheat flour. If you use more, the cake will be too dense.

Store flour in a cool, dry place that is well ventilated. It will absorb odours if stored next to a strongly scented product. If storing flour for a long period of time, it's best to store it in the refrigerator or freezer.

I never sift my flour unless the cake is delicate, as in angel food cakes. The recipe will always say if this is necessary.

sugar

Sugar is used in desserts to provide sweetness and to contribute to the texture of the dessert. It also helps to keep desserts fresh for longer and provides good colour to many desserts, specifically for browning crusts. Its ability to caramelize adds flavour to baked goods.

There are many types of sugar available to the baker. White, dark, light brown, icing, or confectioners sugar and molasses are available. Each type comes from a different stage of the refining process.

White sugar is available in a variety of crystal sizes, from regular granulated to superfine to confectioners or icing sugar. Regular white sugar has larger granules, and icing sugar has very small fine granules.

Icing or confectioners sugar has approximately 3% cornstarch added to each box to prevent lumpiness and crystallization.

brown sugar

Brown sugar is merely white sugar with the addition of molasses. It is less refined than white sugar. The darker the sugar, the more the molasses and moisture it contains. Dark brown sugar is drier and less sweet than light brown sugar. People often think it's a healthier sugar, but it is nutritionally the same as white sugar. The choice is a matter of preference.

Brown sugar tends to make a cake heavier and should be avoided in light-textured cakes. When measuring brown sugar, always pack it firmly.

To avoid lumps from forming in brown sugar, add a slice of old bread to the container and replace it every couple of weeks. Or place the amount of sugar needed in the microwave for 30 seconds, which will help make the sugar more tender.

If you want to make your own brown sugar, add 2 tbsp of unsulphured molasses to 1 cup of granulated sugar.

If you want to cut back on the amount of sugar used in your traditional recipes, as a general rule you can cut about one quarter to one third of the sugar out without affecting the texture. You can cut out more if you use dried or puréed fruit, such as bananas, applesauce, or date purée.

In low-fat baking where fat cannot be used for tenderizing the dessert, sugar is essential for making the dessert tender.

You don't have to sift regular sugar unless it has been sitting for a long time and has developed lumps. Icing sugar should be sifted before using.

sugar substitutes

For those who cannot consume sugar, a sugar replacement is necessary. Some of the sweeteners used in coffee are not ideal, because at high baking temperatures they lose their sweetening power. One of the best on the market is Splenda, which has directions on the box; basically you use one for one. Splenda slightly changes the flavour and texture of a dessert that traditionally uses sugar, but I find it the best substitute.

leavening agents

Leavening agents are added to desserts to make baked goods rise and to produce a light and airy texture. Baking powder and baking soda are the main leaveners used in baking.

baking powder Baking powder is a chemical leavening agent made of acid-reacting materials. There are three main types: single, fast acting or phosphate, and double acting, which is the main one used in home cooking. Baking powder contains approximately 25% cornstarch. The average shelf life of an opened can is about one year. If it is older, it may be the reason your cake is falling.

To test if your baking powder is still fresh, combine 1 tsp baking powder with 1/2 cup hot water; if it bubbles vigorously, it is still fresh. If not, toss it out. Store it in a cool, dark place.

If you run out of baking powder, a good substitution is to combine 2 tsp cream of tartar, 1 tsp baking soda, and a little salt for every cup of flour.

If you use too much baking powder, the cake taste may become bitter, and it may rise rapidly and then collapse.

baking soda Also known as bicarbonate of soda, baking soda is used in baking when there is also an acid, such as buttermilk, yogurt, sour cream, molasses, honey, cocoa, or chocolate. It is needed in order to neutralize some of the acidity, as well as to leaven. Once you add baking soda to the batter, it must be baked immediately or it will begin to rise.

When a recipe calls for both baking soda and baking powder, the baking powder is needed for leavening and the soda neutralizes the acids. Baking soda can darken the colour of chocolate or cocoa in a cake, because it is an alkali.

cream of tartar Cream of tartar is an acidic byproduct of winemaking. It is a white powder used to help prevent the overbeating of egg whites and to help stabilize egg whites during the baking. A mixture that contains cream of tartar should not be cooked in an unlined aluminum pan because the acid reacts with the aluminum and turns the food grey.

salt

Sodium often is confused with the term "salt." Sodium is sodium chloride, a chemical that accounts for 40% of salt. In low-fat baking, often some flavour is removed, therefore a small amount — 1/8 tsp — of salt is often added to enhance the flavours already in the dessert. Salt combines with sugar to bring out and balance the sweetness. I always use it in soy-based desserts, because soy has a flat, bland taste.

cornstarch

Cornstarch is finer than flour and is a more effective thickening agent. As a rule, you use double the flour to cornstarch to thicken a liquid.

gelatin

Gelatin is a natural product derived from collagen, the protein found in bones and connective tissue. Unflavoured gelatin is commonly used in baking and is sold in small boxes that have individual servings of approximately 1 tbsp. Follow the directions on the package, or follow the recipe with specific instructions. The basic principle is to add approximately 2 to 3 tbsp of cold water to 1 tbsp of gelatin and let it sit for 2 minutes to allow the granules to swell; then either heat the mixture in a microwave to melt the gelatin completely or add 2 to 3 tbsp of boiling water and stir until it is combined. Then you add it to your dessert mixture. The dessert may need as long as 2 hours to set properly.

cookie crumbs

Often, to replace a high-fat butter crust, I use cookie crumbs, which have much less fat and fewer calories. My favourites are chocolate wafer crumbs, vanilla wafer crumbs, and graham crumbs. If the cookies have not been ground, just place them whole in a food processor and purée until they are finely ground; then measure what you need. You can even buy your own cookies in bulk and do the same thing.

The reason these crusts are lower in fat is because they are held together mostly with water and just a small amount of fat.

quick-cooking oats

I like to use quick-cooking oats in baking because they give desserts texture, taste, and volume without adding fat and calories. Be sure to use either quick-cooking or old-fashioned rolled oats. Do not use instant oats, because they tend to make the batter sticky.

liquids

sweeteners

honey Honey lends a specific flavour and baking quality to pastries. It's best to use it only when called for. Honey is sweeter and has a higher moisture content than granulated sugar. As a rule, use one third less honey than sugar and when possible reduce the volume of other liquids by 1/4 cup for each cup of honey used.

corn syrup Corn syrup is made when starch granules are extracted from corn kernels and treated with acid to break them down into a sweet syrup. It comes from the glucose from the corn sugar plus some added fructose and water. It is great in low-fat baking because it can replicate some qualities of oil.

  I prefer light corn syrup for these recipes. Before measuring corn syrup, slightly grease the measuring cup so the corn syrup will pour out easily.

molasses Molasses is the liquid separated from sugar crystals during the first stages of refining sugar. Its colour and strength depend on the stage of the separation process. The first liquid molasses drawn off is the finest quality, the second and later ones contain more impurities. The third is called blackstrap, which is the blackest and has the strongest flavour. For baking, select the dark molasses.

maple syrup Pure maple syrup comes from the sap of the sugar maple tree, which is boiled down until it has evaporated and thickened. It takes about 30 gallons of maple sap to produce 1 gallon of syrup. That's why the cost is so high for pure syrup. I like to buy Grade A or Fancy Grade syrup, which is light brown in colour and has a delicious delicate flavour. It is quite expensive but it is well worth the cost. Try to avoid imitation maple syrups, which are basically corn syrup with artificial maple flavouring and colour added.

juices

Always use fresh lemon or lime juice. The bottled versions have a bitter aftertaste and are only fine if the fruit juice is not the predominant flavour in the dessert. I often squeeze more juice than I need and pour it into ice cube trays and freeze. Then pop out the cubes and store them in airtight plastic bags so they're available when you need them. One lemon produces approximately 1/3 cup juice and 1 lime approximately 1/4 cup juice. One orange yields approximately 1/2 cup juice.

For orange juice, I'll use fresh if I've used the rind; otherwise I find the concentrates or those bottled or sold in cartons are fine for baking purposes. I use orange juice concentrate a lot because of the intensity of flavour. I keep a can in the freezer just for baking and cooking purposes.

coffee

I like the taste of coffee in some of my desserts. Either use instant coffee or a strong brew. I always use a higher ration of dry instant to water than would be called for drinking. Instant espresso powder is available in some groceries and produces a more intense flavour than regular instant coffee powder (but less caffeine!).

fats

Baking fats include butter, margarine, vegetable shortening, lard, and oil. For low-fat baking. I use only butter, margarine, or oil. Fats in baking tenderize, moisturize, add flakiness, and add flavour. They also add a smoother texture to the dessert.

Fats are either saturated or unsaturated. Unsaturated fats are liquid at room temperature, such as oil. Saturated fats are solid, such as butter, lard, and some margarine. Better-quality margarine is mostly unsaturated fat.

Doughs containing butter or margarine soften in the oven and spread quickly. Cookies, for example, are thin and crisp. Shortening cookies stay thicker because they set before the fat melts.

For the recipes in this book, you can use oil, butter, or margarine interchangeably, without losing texture or flavour.

butter

Butter has the best flavour of all fats. For cooking, it should always be unsalted. Keep in mind that butter is an animal fat so it contains cholesterol, and it is saturated. Too much saturated fat leads to excess weight and increased cholesterol in one's blood, which can lead to heart and circulatory problems.

margarine

Margarine was invented by a French chemist in the late 19th century to provide an inexpensive fat for the army of Napoleon III. It is made from a variety of oils and solid fats that are mixed and heated. We are taught that we should only consume margarines with the least amount of saturated fats and the most amount of monounsaturated fats. Choose soft-tub margarine, not hard. The total grams of polyunsaturated and monounsaturated fat should be no more than 6 g. Never use calorie-reduced margarine for baking. It's always best to keep your fat intake to a minimum and not worry about the type of fat used if you're only using small amounts.

Because certain margarines can be hydrogenated, which turns them into a form of saturated fat, I prefer to use either oil or butter, or a combination of the two.

vegetable oils

All vegetable oils have approximately the same amount of calories and fat. Vegetable oils contain no cholesterol. They contain different amounts of polyunsaturated and monounsaturated fats. Oils high in polyunsaturated fats include safflower, sunflower, corn, soy, and cottonseed. These fats can help to lower the "bad" (LDL) cholesterol in one's blood.

Monounsaturated oils are the most desirable. They include canola oil, peanut oil, and olive oil.

vegetable oil spray

I like to use vegetable oil spray to coat my baking pans, because it is a convenient and low-fat way to keep baked desserts from sticking to the pan. Sprays are usually a mixture of oil and lecithin. I prefer a canola spray. Most of the sprays such as Pam contain canola oil, grain alcohol, and butter flavouring. You can also fill a spray pump bottle halfway with vegetable oil and use this to spray your pans.

fat substitutes

I don't buy artificial fat substitutes. Instead, the substitutes I work with are all natural. Using cooked or fresh fruit purées is one technique. Puréed ripe bananas give great texture and flavour to a dessert. Applesauce and purées made of cooked dried fruits such as dates, prunes, apricots, and figs are also wonderful. The rule is that you can successfully reduce the fat in a traditional recipe by as much as 75% and substitute the above. You must have some fat for flavour, texture, and shelf life — so don't omit all the fat.

Another technique is to use grated vegetables, such as carrots, beets, and zucchini, which also help to add moisture and texture that fat can add.

Low-fat sour cream, yogurt, and buttermilk also help to maintain texture and flavour, while greatly reducing the fat.

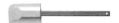

eggs

Eggs are very important in baking. They add richness and nutrition in the form of proteins, vitamins, and minerals, and they add to the texture, colour, and flavour of your dessert. They also help bind a batter together: when a cake rises during baking, the proteins in the eggs combine with the proteins in the flour to keep the structure stable.

One whole egg contains 75 calories, of which over 60% come from fat. The yolk contains all the fat and the cholesterol. I like to use some whole eggs in my recipes not only for the taste but also for the texture. I am careful not to use too many due to the fat and cholesterol they contain. Often I combine 1 whole egg and 2 egg whites in a dessert. The white has no fat or cholesterol and 1 egg white only contains 15 calories and 3.5 g of protein. It still helps bind the batter.

If you want to substitute a whole egg with egg whites, use 2 whites for every whole egg. But remember that too many egg whites can make a cake batter too dry. I often use 1 whole egg to balance the flavour and texture.

Don't get too concerned about the fat and cholesterol of the egg yolk, because that one yolk, which may have 5 g of fat, is being divided among the entire dessert, which may produce up to 12 servings.

In many of my recipes I am able to reduce the fat, calories, and cholesterol greatly not only by adding more egg whites but also by whipping them with cream of tartar, which helps to stabilize them, and with sugar to sweeten. This combination adds a greater volume to the dessert without adding fat. See "Beating Egg Whites" on page 21 for tips.

safety of meringues

I once filmed an episode of my cooking show at an egg factory. The management informed me that only 1 in every 20,000 eggs will contain salmonella bacteria. Chances are this one egg is found in restaurants or establishments that work with lots of eggs and leave them out at room temperature for hours. Usually in your home, your eggs are refrigerated. I don't worry about salmonella in my home. But if you are concerned, here is what you can do.

An egg must be cooked to a temperature of 140°F for 3 1/2 minutes or 150°F for 2 minutes. If you are beating egg whites, you can follow the recipe for Italian meringue. You combine 2 to 3 egg whites with 1/4 tsp cream of tartar, 1/4 cup water, and 1/4 to 1/2 cup sugar in the top of a double boiler. Keep the water simmering and beat the egg white mixture for approximately 6 to 8 minutes or until the meringue is glossy and smooth and holds its shape. Remove it from the double boiler and continue beating for 1 minute. Use a stainless steel bowl, which heats faster than a glass bowl. This meringue is more stable than regular meringues.

storing eggs

Egg whites can be refrigerated for up to a month. Egg yolks can be refrigerated in a covered jar for 2 to 3 days. Put a drop of water over the yolks to keep them moist. To freeze leftover eggs, stir and blend them with a few grains of salt or sugar and freeze in ice cube trays. One cube equals one egg. They can be frozen for up to 1 year. Thaw them overnight in the refrigerator before using and never refreeze thawed eggs.

egg whites

You're probably using more egg whites than yolks. Rather than tossing out the yolks, giving them to your dogs, or saving them for a special rich dessert, you can buy egg whites in a container at most grocery stores. One large egg white equals 2 tbsp of the liquid in the container. Four large egg whites equal 1/2 cup. They also make great egg-white omelettes.

egg substitutes

I prefer not to use chemically based egg substitutes. There are different egg substitutes on the market that try to duplicate the flavour and texture of egg yolks, without the fat and cholesterol. Read the ingredients thoroughly to make sure it's not a synthetic product. Many use a host of additives and preservatives including monosodium glutamate (MSG), artificial flavour, colouring, and modified food starches. There are some natural products that mix 20% yolks to 80% whites and taste delicious without additives.

milk and milk products

With most milk products, I like to use the low-fat versions. I save a lot of calories, fat, and cholesterol, and, because of all the other flavours in the desserts, I don't feel any taste or texture is missed. Judge for yourself.

I always use either 1% or 2% MF (milk fat).

calories and fat of milk products

1 cup of **whole milk**, which is 3.5% MF, has 150 calories and 8 g of fat.

2% MF milk is 125 calories per cup with 5 g of fat; 1% milk has 119 calories and 3 g of fat; and skim milk has 99 calories and 2 g of fat.

Buttermilk has 99 calories and 2 g of fat per cup.

Evaporated skim milk has 199 calories and 1 g of fat per cup, compared to evaporated whole milk, which has 338 calories per cup and 19 g of fat.

Sweetened condensed milk has 983 calories per cup with 27 g of fat versus low-fat condensed milk, which has 960 calories and 12 g of fat per cup.

Sour cream has 493 calories per cup with 48 g of fat, compared to low-fat sour cream, which has 360 calories and 28 g of fat. Fat-free sour cream has 360 calories per cup with 0 g of fat.

Low-fat yogurt has 144 calories per cup with 4 g of fat and non-fat yogurt has 127 calories with 0 g of fat.

2 tbsp of **full-fat cream cheese** have 100 calories and 10 g of fat versus the 50% less-fat version, which has 70 calories and 5 g of fat per 2 tbsp.

Ricotta cheese with whole milk has 432 calories and 32 g of fat per cup. The lighter version has 340 calories and 20 g of fat.

Cottage cheese with whole milk has 217 calories and 10 g of fat per cup. Cottage cheese with 1% MF has 164 calories and 2 g of fat per cup.

buttermilk

Buttermilk is made by letting bacteria in regular milk thicken and create a tangy taste. It creates a fat-like texture without the fat, calories, and cholesterol. You can make your own by adding 1 tbsp lemon juice to 1 cup milk and letting it stand for 5 minutes.

canned evaporated milk

Evaporated milk either comes in whole fat, 2% MF, and skim. It is milk with 60% of the water removed. It has a thicker texture than regular milk and has a sweeter flavour. I often use it in place of heavy cream or whole milk in a recipe. It creates a thick, rich texture and creamier taste. Two table-spoons of regular canned milk contain 40 calories with 2.5 g of fat. The skim milk version has 25 calories and 0 g of fat.

sweetened condensed milk

Sweetened condensed milk is a mixture of milk and sugar. The milk is heated until about 60% of the water evaporates, producing an extremely sticky and sweet milk, perfect in desserts to add thickness and sweetness. It is approximately 45% sugar. Fortunately, it now exists in a low-fat version. Two tablespoons of regular condensed milk contain 130 calories and 3 g of fat. The low-fat version has 120 calories and only 1.5 g of fat.

yogurt

Yogurt is a nutritious, low-fat, low-cholesterol product containing high levels of calcium, protein, and B vitamins. It is made from skim milk that is homogenized, pasteurized, and injected with live bacteria, including the most valuable bacteria, *Lactobacillus acidophilus*. These bacteria feed on the milk sugar to produce lactic acid. The milk is then allowed to ferment in order to coagulate into yogurt and develop that characteristic tangy flavour.

There are all different fat contents of yogurt. I usually prefer 1% MF. For a creamier texture use 2% MF yogurt. Most recipes call for plain unflavoured yogurt. The flavoured yogurts are available in 1% MF or lower. I prefer to use those with sugar rather than a sugar substitute.

Low-fat yogurt is a good substitute for sour cream or heavy cream. I often use it interchangeably with low-fat sour cream.

sour cream

Sour cream is basically fermented heavy cream. It's made from 18% butterfat cream that has been injected with bacteria and allowed to thicken. Fortunately, there are now low-fat sour creams available with anywhere from 5% MF or lower. I even use fat-free sour cream in my baking and don't know the difference.

cream cheese

Cream cheese made from milk must contain at least 33% butterfat and has 100 calories per ounce. Fortunately, today there is light cream cheese, which is 25% reduced in fat. This is not a considerable difference, but it is good enough to use light cream cheese to highlight my recipes. I will not depend on the cream cheese to make the recipe. For instance, I use a combination of either ricotta or cottage cheese along with a small amount of cream cheese. The light cream cheese gives the dessert a smoother texture and delicate flavour.

Be careful not to use the soft light cream cheese in the tub. It does not have the same properties for baking and should not be substituted. In the United States there is fat-free cream cheese. I find its taste and texture inferior. Do not bake with it.

cottage cheese

Cottage cheese is a fresh, unripened cheese — one of the oldest cheeses known to humans. It is white and has small or large curds.

A wide variety of cottage cheeses is available, from 4% MF right down to 1% MF. I find that either 1% or 2% MF is best to use in desserts. If you replace ricotta with cottage cheese, remember to purée it well to smooth the curds. I don't like to use dry curd cottage cheese because the texture is too dry. If you do use it, however, add some milk to smooth it out.

ricotta cheese

In North America, ricotta cheese is made from whole milk or a combination of milk and whey. Ricotta cheese that is fresh and unripened has fine moist clumps and a bland but almost nutty taste. Italian ricotta cheese is made from sheep's milk drained from the curds when provolone cheese is made.

The regular fat content is approximately 10%, but now there is 5% MF available. Low-fat ricotta cheese is made from skim milk. I don't find a difference in baking when I use the 5% MF.

I always look for a creamy smooth ricotta cheese, not one that has been dried and pressed. If you only have the dry-pressed ricotta cheese, add 2 tbsp of water or milk and mix until it is smooth.

Because ricotta is a fresh cheese, it doesn't have a long shelf life and should be used within a few days. It can be frozen for baking purposes, which changes the texture slightly.

I use ricotta cheese in many desserts to replace some of the fat or cream cheese that may have been used traditionally.

soy products

For the soy section, I used low-fat soy milk, silken tofu, or firm tofu. These products are perfect for those who have milk allergies, are lactose intolerant, are vegetarian, or are kosher. Soy is easy to digest, is low in calories, cholesterol, and sodium, and is high in protein.

Look at the soy section beginning on page 154 for tips on using soy in your desserts.

passover products

During Passover, all wheat flour products and any leavening agents must be avoided. There are many excellent products during Passover that can be used for baking. The main substitute for flour is matzo cake meal with a combination of potato starch. Look at the section on Passover beginning on page 172 for more detail.

flavourings and spices

Spices, extracts, citrus rind or zest, liqueurs, coffee, and chocolate all add incredible flavour to your desserts, especially low-fat desserts, since you can't just rely on the butter, cream, or pounds of chocolate!

spices

Once a spice is ground, its aroma fades quickly if it is exposed to air or heat or if it is around for a long period of time. Keep your spices in tightly closed jars and replace them every 6 months.

extracts

Pure extracts are the concentrated natural essential oils of the flavouring agent, usually dissolved in alcohol. They are labelled either "pure" or "artificial." Only buy the pure. It's more expensive, but well worth the expense. I find the artificial extracts usually leave a bitter aftertaste in the dessert.

rind

Rind or zest is the brightly coloured part of the peel of a citrus fruit. In my recipes, I call for lemon, lime, or orange rind. The rind contains the fruit's essential flavours. Be careful not to grate too much or you'll get the white pith under the rind, which will make the dessert bitter. I like to use a citrus peeler — a kitchen gadget with a flat metal head containing five tiny sharp-edged holes. It makes grating the fruit easy and safe.

One lemon yields approximately 1 tbsp of zest, 1 lime approximately 2 tsp, and 1 orange approximately 2 tbsp.

dried fruit

I use a wide variety of dried fruits in these desserts — dried dates, prunes, apricots, figs, cherries, raisins, cranberries, and more. They add flavour and their natural sugar provides sweetness. Dried fruits are also a great nutritional boost, because they are a valuable source of vitamins, minerals, and fibre.

Cooked and puréed dried fruit supplies an alternative to some of the fat used in the recipe. I often replace up to 75% of the fat in a recipe with cooked puréed dried fruit. Don't try to replace all the fat with fruit purées or your dessert will be too dry, lack flavour, and will not have a long shelf life.

To make your own fruit purée, cut up the dried fruit and measure 1 cup. Add 1 cup of water and cook over medium-low heat, taking care that enough liquid remains to prevent scorching, until the fruit is soft. Then purée the fruit in a food processor until it is smooth.

Be sure to buy pitted dried fruit. The easiest way to chop these fruits is with scissors. I buy them in bulk and keep them in the freezer.

nuts

I love to use nuts to highlight my desserts. Keep in mind they contain a lot of calories and fat, but it is the healthy type of fat — either polyunsaturated or monounsaturated fat. Toasting nuts brings out their flavour. To do this, just add nuts to a skillet on a high heat and toast, stirring constantly, for approximately 2 to 3 minutes or until the nuts begin to brown. Then either use them as they are or chop them to the desired consistency in a food processor.

If a traditional recipe calls for a lot of nuts, try using only 25% of the original amount and replacing the remainder with Grape-Nuts, which is a delicious toasted wheat and barley breakfast cereal that is a great low-fat substitute for nuts.

chocolate and cocoa

I prefer to buy chocolate in chips rather than in blocks of chocolate. It is easier to measure and to melt. The 1-oz squares are fine to use, too. The chocolate must be stored in a dry cool place and can last for years. It may develop a white surface over time, which means that the cocoa butter has risen to the surface. It is still good to use.

types of chocolate

semi-sweet and bitter Both semi-sweet and bitter chocolates contain vanilla, sugar, and cocoa butter. In my recipes I only use semi-sweet, which has a wonderful sweet and creamy taste and texture.

milk Dry milk is added to sweetened chocolate to create milk chocolate. I use milk chocolate chips in some desserts.

white White chocolate is not true chocolate because it does not contain chocolate liquor and has very little chocolate flavour, but it is nonetheless mouth watering. It contains cocoa butter, sugar, and milk. I like to use white chocolate chips to highlight some of the desserts.

compound or baking chocolate This is an artificial chocolate that's best used for decorations. It contains vegetable fat instead of cocoa butter. Don't use it in the recipes, or you'll end up with no chocolate flavour.

melting chocolate

A good way to melt chocolate is to place it in a bowl in the microwave and heat at either medium or high (only if you're confident). One ounce of chocolate chips equals 2 tbsp and will take approximately 1 minute at high or 2 minutes at medium to melt. How long depends on how much cocoa butter the chocolate contains. Always err on the side of being conservative — it is better to add more cooking time than to burn the chocolate, which often cannot be salvaged. Just heat the chocolate until it appears to melt and then stir it until it's smooth.

One of the safest ways is to use the traditional double boiler method. Place the chocolate in the top of the double boiler over a simmering heat. Remove the top pot when the chocolate begins to melt. Stir until it is smooth.

Be careful when melting white chocolate, which tends to solidify easily and can turn lumpy. I would use a lower heat in the microwave, and use it immediately after melting.

If a little water accidentally touches your melted chocolate, it will seize up. If this happens, add 1 tsp of vegetable oil and stir quickly. Chocolate can be melted with another liquid such as water or coffee when the correct amount in the recipe is added.

cocoa

Cocoa is made when chocolate liquor is pressed to remove over half the cocoa butter. One ounce of cocoa has approximately 60 calories and 4 g of fat, compared to chocolate, which has 130 calories and 9 g of fat per oz. This is the reason I use cocoa in all my chocolate desserts, and occasionally I highlight the dessert with either chocolate chips or a little melted chocolate.

equipment
baking pans

Here is a list of the pans I recommend for your kitchen:
- three 8-inch round and square metal nonstick pans
- three 9-inch round and square metal nonstick pans

- one 9-inch × 13-inch nonstick baking pan
- two 8-inch springform pans
- two 9-inch springform pans
- two 10-inch springform pans
- two 9-inch nonstick Bundt pans
- one 10-inch nonstick tube pan with removable bottom
- three 9-inch glass pie plates
- two 15-inch × 10-inch jelly roll pans
- two 9-inch × 5-inch loaf pans
- two 8-inch tart pans with removable bottom
- two 9-inch tart pans with removable bottom
- eight 6-oz ovenproof ramekins or custard cups
- three large nonstick baking sheets
- small, medium, and large nonstick saucepans
- small, medium, and large nonstick skillets

Baking pans can be made of metal or glass, but cakes bake slightly faster in glass pans. I always recommend checking your baked desserts 5 to 10 minutes before the specified baking time, due to different qualities of pans and differences in oven temperatures.

utensils and special equipment

- Assorted mixing bowls
- Metal and plastic spatulas and whisks
- Knives — chefs, slicing, serrated
- Wooden spoons
- Measuring cups for liquids and dry ingredients
- Measuring spoons
- Scale
- Zester
- Parchment paper
- Wooden or metal cake testers

electric equipment

There are a wide variety of electric mixers available today. Kitchen Aid is a popular brand and the one I used on my television show. The wire whisk or flat paddle-type beater is used most for all general-purpose cake baking. However, because low-fat baking doesn't require creaming butter, sugar, and eggs, I don't find this piece of equipment very necessary. I generally use a food processor, beater, and whisk for all my baking.

I love food processors, but they must be treated with respect. I recommend one with two bowls and two metal blades for mixing cakes, chopping nuts, making cookie crumb crusts, and blending mixtures. I only use the metal blade. Wet ingredients cannot be overbeaten, but be careful not to overbeat the flour. Once the flour and other dry ingredients are added to the wet, you should use the pulse or on/off feature just until the flour is incorporated. Then with a wooden spoon mix until everything is well blended. Overmixing will toughen your cake or cookies.

Electric beaters are great for beating egg whites and mixing ingredients in general.

ovens

Each oven is different. If I use three different ovens, I get different times and results each time. Know your oven well, whether it's electric, gas, or convection. I have to be honest. I use an electric oven and get great results every time — because I always check the dessert 5 to 10 minutes before the specified baking time.

Convection ovens are ideal for baking cheesecakes because they distribute the heat evenly throughout the oven. As a general rule, reduce the recommended temperature by 25°F to 50°F and the recommended baking time by 20% to 30%. But you must always check the dessert.

Know your oven's hot spots. I prefer to bake in the middle of the oven, to get the best overall results. Have your oven checked every two years, because the temperatures can fluctuate with use. Most ovens are off by at least 25°F, which naturally affects the results. Always check your baked dessert 5 to 10 minutes before the time in the recipe is up, just to be sure.

Don't open the door before you check the dessert. Cold air can cause a cake to fall or crack. When a cake is done, the colour of the top should often be golden brown, the edges should just begin to pull away from the sides, and the dessert cake should appear firm, not loose. Always use a cake tester and insert it into the centre. It should come out clean and dry.

microwave oven

For baking, I use a microwave only to defrost, melt, or warm. I don't bake my desserts here.

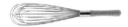

special techniques for desserts

measuring

When measuring dry ingredients, always level them off with a knife. When measuring liquid ingredients, use measuring cups suited for liquid ingredients.

beating, blending, and whisking

Beating, blending, and whisking are all ways to mix ingredients rapidly either with a whisk, wooden spoon, or electric mixer. Blending is stirring or mixing ingredients until they are well combined. Whisking means to beat ingredients with a hand-held whisk until the ingredients are mixed completely.

beating egg whites

The trick to beating egg whites properly is to use a clean bowl and clean beaters. Use a hand beater or an electric mixer with a large balloon beater. I find egg whites at room temperature beat best and to the greatest volume. They tend to separate best when cold. If there is any foreign material in your bowl, especially fat (perhaps from a drop of egg yolk) or even water, the egg whites will not beat, no matter how long you beat them. To get rid of any grease in a bowl, wipe it with a paper towel dampened with white vinegar. Avoid plastic bowls when beating egg whites, because they can never be cleaned completely of grease residue.

There is one way you might salvage the egg whites. Try adding 2 tsp of lemon juice to every 2 egg whites. This sometimes helps to beat them properly. If this fails, you'll have to try again with fresh egg whites, but with clean and dry bowls and beaters.

To beat egg whites, begin beating them with a bit of cream of tartar until they are foamy; gradually add the sugar and keep beating until the whites are glossy and smooth. Be sure that the sugar granules are completely dissolved in the egg whites, especially for meringues, which will "weep" during baking when undissolved sugar granules melt and ooze out. To test if the sugar is dissolved, pinch some of the beaten egg whites between your thumb and forefinger. If it feels grainy, the sugar granules are still whole; if it is smooth, the sugar is dissolved. Continue beating until stiff peaks almost form. You should be able to turn the bowl upside down without the whites losing their shape. At this point, the egg whites are stiff but not dry. Avoid overbeating the whites, or you'll destroy the texture: the whites will become lumpy and dry and they'll move with liquid at the bottom of the bowl. You can salvage overbeaten whites by adding one more egg white to the beaten ones and beating again.

folding

Folding egg whites into the batter must be done correctly to maintain volume in the mixture. Use a rubber spatula and insert the lighter mixture into the middle of the bowl containing the heavier mixture; drag it down through the mixture toward you, gently scraping the bottom of the bowl and lifting the mixture from the bottom to the top. Just be careful of overfolding, because you can deflate the whites and end up with a poor volume.

water bath or bain marie

A water bath or bain marie is a large pan of water into which you place your dessert pan. This allows the dessert to bake more evenly and keeps the texture smoother. It is often used with custards, brûlées, crème caramels, soufflés, and pudding cakes.

When baking cheesecakes, I like to place a pan of water on the lowest rack to prevent the cheesecake from cracking and make more moisture in the oven to keep the consistency of the cheesecake smooth.

cooling cakes

Remove the pan from the oven, set it on a cooling rack away from cold air for approximately 15 to 20 minutes. Loosen the sides of the cake from the pan with a knife. Then invert the cake onto the rack and let it cool completely before icing or placing in the refrigerator or freezer. This method often prevents cracking, especially with cheesecakes.

ingredients at room temperature

Every cookbook says ingredients should be at room temperature. I confess that I don't always follow this rule because I'm often in a hurry. But ingredients are easier to incorporate when they are at room temperature.

freezing cakes and desserts

Many desserts can be frozen and stored for later use. After the cake has cooled on the wire rack, wrap it in plastic wrap or foil and place it inside a freezer plastic bag. Make sure you get as much of the air out of the bag as possible. You can freeze an iced cake by first placing it on a baking sheet in the freezer until the icing is firm, approximately 20 minutes. Then wrap as stated above.

To thaw cakes, leave them wrapped until they thaw out, in the refrigerator.

Do not freeze custards, brûlées, soufflés, desserts made with cottage cheese, or those with a lot of beaten egg whites.

nutritional information

All the recipes in this book have been analyzed for calories, fat, saturated fat, cholesterol, carbohydrates, and fibre. The recipes were analyzed using canola oil, soft-tub margarine, 1% MF yogurt, 1% MF, 5% MF ricotta, and 2% MF cottage cheese. The nutritional package is from ESHA Research's Food Processor Nutrition Analysis Software and Databases.

Before examining the nutritional analysis for each recipe, let's look at the chart below and see what the nutritional daily recommendations are for men and women aged 25 to 50:

	Women	Men
Calories	2000	2700
Fat	67 g or less	90 g or less
Saturated fat	22 g or less	30 g or less
Carbohydrates	299 g	405 g
Fibre	25–35 g	25–35 g
Cholesterol	300 mg or less	300 mg or less

Now check out the recipe you're preparing and see how it compares to your recommended daily total. You'll be surprised to see how low in calories, fat, and cholesterol these delicious desserts are, and how well they fit daily into a healthy diet. Having one piece of delicious dessert is not only allowed every day — I recommend it!

Let's also compare a high-fat cheesecake to one of my low-fat versions. For example, this chart compares a typical piece of my cheesecake with a regular one.

	Low-fat cheesecake	High-fat cheesecake
Calories	250	640
Total fat	7 g	32 g
Saturated fat	3 g	22 g
Carbohydrates	30 g	40 g
Cholesterol	40 mg	120 mg
Fibre	1 g	1 g

In summary, one cannot afford the calories, fat, and cholesterol of high-fat desserts on a daily basis without gaining weight or harming health. With my low-fat desserts, there is no reason you cannot enjoy dessert every day.

layer cakes

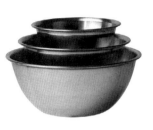

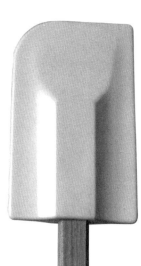

tips for divine light layer cakes

1. Layer cakes are baked in 8- or 9-inch round or square pans. Always spray the pans with vegetable spray. It doesn't matter if you use glass or metal pans, but check the baking times because glass may cook faster.

2. If you use a different size pan than the recipe calls for, adjust the baking time accordingly. A cake baked in a 8-inch pan takes more time than one in a 9-inch pan (add or subtract 10 minutes per inch).

3. Always preheat the oven and have all the ingredients on hand. It's better to have ingredients at room temperature.

4. Place the pan in the centre of the oven and check for doneness by inserting a toothpick or tester into the centre of the cake. The cake is done when the tester comes out dry and clean.

5. Cool cakes on racks until they are at room temperature. Then invert them onto racks before icing.

6. A good way to ice a layer cake is to use a springform: place one layer in the pan, ice the middle, then place the other layer cake over top. Let the pan sit in the freezer for 10 minutes to prevent the icing from coming out the sides. Then ice the entire cake.

7. Italian meringue icing is a delicious low-fat icing made by beating egg whites with sugar and water over a very low heat. This process kills any bacteria in the egg whites and makes an icing that lasts much longer and is more stable than regular meringue toppings. Use it with any cake or muffin recipe. You can create a variety of icings by adding flavourings such as almond extract, orange juice concentrate, or cocoa.

lemon poppyseed cake with lemon curd filling

Lemon, lemon, and more lemon. That's my definition of divine. Orange juice gives the lemon curd a rich colour because no butter is used.

LEMON CURD
2/3 cup orange juice
2 tsp finely grated lemon rind
1/3 cup fresh lemon juice
1 cup granulated sugar
1/4 cup cornstarch

CAKE
1 1/4 cups granulated sugar
1/3 cup vegetable oil
1 large egg
1 large egg white
2 tsp finely grated lemon rind
1/4 cup fresh lemon juice
2 tsp poppyseeds

1 1/3 cups all-purpose flour
1 1/2 tsp baking powder
1/2 tsp baking soda
2/3 cup low-fat sour cream
2 large egg whites
1/4 tsp cream of tartar
3 tbsp granulated sugar

Preheat the oven to 350°F. Spray two 9-inch round cake pans with vegetable spray.

1. Make lemon curd: In a small saucepan off the heat, whisk together orange juice, lemon rind and juice, sugar, and cornstarch until smooth. Cook over medium heat, whisking constantly, for 8 minutes or until the mixture is clear, thickened, and bubbling. Transfer the mixture to a bowl. Place a piece of plastic wrap directly on surface of lemon curd. Chill the curd while you prepare the cakes.
2. Make cake: In a large bowl and using a whisk or electric mixer, beat 1 1/4 cups sugar, oil, egg, egg white, lemon rind, lemon juice, and poppyseeds.
3. In another bowl, stir together flour, baking powder, and baking soda. With a wooden spoon, stir them into the sugar mixture in batches, alternating with sour cream, just until combined.
4. In another bowl, beat egg whites with cream of tartar until they are foamy. Gradually add 3 tbsp sugar, beating until stiff peaks form. Stir one quarter of egg whites into the cake batter. Gently fold in remaining egg whites just until blended. Divide the mixture between the prepared pans.
5. Bake in the centre of the oven for 18 to 20 minutes or until a tester comes out dry.
6. Let the pans cool on a wire rack.
7. Place one cake layer on a cake platter. Spread some curd over top. Place the second cake layer on top of the first and top with the remaining curd.

MAKES 14 SERVINGS

NUTRITIONAL ANALYSIS
PER SERVING
Energy 270 calories
Protein 3 g
Fat, total 6.6 g
Fat, saturated 1.1 g
Carbohydrates 49 g
Fibre 0.5 g
Cholesterol 18 mg

NUTRITION WATCH
Lemons are an excellent source of vitamin C, but they start to lose their vitamin power soon after being squeezed.

TIP
To get the most volume when beating egg whites, always use a clean and dry bowl and beaters. Any foreign substance will prevent the whites from foaming. If this does happen, try adding 2 tsp lemon juice for every 2 egg whites and continue beating.

banana poppyseed layer cake with chocolate icing

MAKES 14 SERVINGS

NUTRITIQNAL ANALYSIS
PER SERVING
Energy 269 calories
Protein 5.4 g
Fat, total 8.4 g
Fat, saturated 2.1 g
Carbohydrates 42 g
Fibre 1.3 g
Cholesterol 24 mg

NUTRITION WATCH
Bananas are loaded with
potassium and are an excellent source of carbohydrates
and vitamin C. Enjoy them as
a nutritious snack any time
of the day.

TIP
You can substitute low-fat
sour cream for the yogurt.
Either product comes in
1% MF or less.

Bananas and chocolate make an incredible combination in a dessert. The ripeness of the bananas gives this cake lots of flavour. I keep my overripe bananas in the freezer so I can thaw them to use in any dish requiring puréed bananas.

CAKE
1/3 cup vegetable oil
1 large egg
1 large egg white
1 large (1/2 cup) ripe banana,
    mashed
2 tsp vanilla
1 cup granulated sugar
2 tsp poppyseeds
1 1/4 cups all-purpose flour

2 tsp baking powder
1/2 tsp baking soda
2/3 cup low-fat yogurt

ICING
2 oz light cream cheese, softened
1 cup smooth 5% ricotta cheese
1 1/2 cups icing sugar
1/4 cup unsweetened cocoa powder
1 small ripe banana

Preheat the oven to 350°F. Spray two 9-inch round cake pans with vegetable spray.

1. Make cake: In a large bowl and using a whisk or electric mixer, beat oil, egg, egg white, banana, vanilla, sugar, and poppyseeds.

2. In another bowl, stir together flour, baking powder, and baking soda. With a wooden spoon, stir the dry ingredients into the poppyseed mixture in batches, alternating with yogurt, just until combined. Divide the mixture between the prepared pans.

3. Place the pans in the centre of the oven and bake for 15 to 20 minutes or until a tester inserted in the centre comes out dry.

4. Let the pans cool on a wire rack.

5. Make icing: In a food processor, beat cream cheese, ricotta cheese, icing sugar, and cocoa until the mixture is smooth.

6. Place one cake layer on a cake platter. Spread icing over top. Slice the banana and place the slices on the cake layer. Place the second cake layer on top and ice the top and sides.

banana chocolate fudge layer cake

I don't know anyone who doesn't love the combination of banana and chocolate.
This layer cake is divinely moist and tender — even the icing is lovely and light.

MAKES 12 SERVINGS

NUTRITIONAL ANALYSIS
PER SERVING
Energy 265 calories
Protein 8 g
Fat, total 9 g
Fat, saturated 3 g
Carbohydrates 39 g
Sodium 241 mg
Fibre 2 g
Cholesterol 42 mg

BANANA CAKE
3 tbsp margarine or butter
1/3 cup granulated sugar
1 large egg
1 large (1/2 cup) ripe
   banana, mashed
1 tsp vanilla
3/4 cup all-purpose flour
1/2 tsp baking soda
1/4 cup low-fat yogurt

CHOCOLATE
FUDGE CAKE
3 tbsp margarine or butter
3/4 cup brown sugar
1 large egg
3 tbsp unsweetened cocoa
   powder
1/2 cup all-purpose flour
1/2 tsp baking soda
1/2 tsp baking powder
1/3 cup low-fat yogurt

FROSTING
1 1/2 cups 5% smooth
   ricotta cheese
1 cup icing sugar
1/4 cup unsweetened cocoa
   powder
Half banana

Preheat the oven to 350°F. Spray two 8-inch round cake pans with vegetable spray.

1. Make banana cake: Combine margarine and sugar in a large bowl or food processor; mix until smooth. Add egg, banana, and vanilla; mix until everything is well combined. In a small bowl, stir together flour and baking soda; add the flour mixture to the banana mixture in batches, alternating with the yogurt, just until combined. Pour the mixture into a prepared pan.

2. Make chocolate fudge cake: Combine margarine, sugar, and egg in a large bowl; mix until everything is well combined (the mixture may look curdled). In a small bowl, stir together cocoa, flour, baking soda, and baking powder; add the mixture to the batter in batches, alternating with the yogurt, just until combined. Pour mixture into a prepared pan.

3. Place both pans in the centre of the oven and bake for 15 to 20 minutes or until a tester inserted in the centre comes out clean.

4. Make frosting: In a bowl and using a food processor or electric mixer, beat ricotta cheese, icing sugar, and cocoa until smooth.

5. Assemble cake: Put the banana cake on a cake platter; top with one quarter of the frosting. Thinly slice the banana and place slices over top. Put the chocolate cake on top and use the remaining frosting to frost the sides and top.

NUTRITION WATCH
This layer cake is light because it uses puréed bananas and low-fat sour cream to reduce the fat content, and the icing uses low-fat yogurt instead of butter or other shortening.

TIPS
This makes a heavenly birthday cake. It's delicious — and healthier than most. For a special effect, double the recipe and create a four-layer extravaganza. The ricotta cheese gives the icing its smooth butter-like texture.

Eliminate the cocoa for white icing. You may have to cut back on the icing sugar, though.

sour cream chocolate cake

MAKES 16 SERVINGS

NUTRITIONAL ANALYSIS
PER SERVING
Energy 256 calories
Protein 3.6 g
Fat, total 8.6 g
Fat, saturated 2.8 g
Carbohydrates 41 g
Fibre 1.7 g
Cholesterol 37 mg

NUTRITION WATCH
Substitute low-fat sour cream
1% MF or less for regular
sour cream, which has
14% MF, in all your recipes.
The texture and taste remain
excellent.

TIP
You can use 0% MF sour
cream, which has a fine texture for cakes and icing.

With its sour cream topping, this rich and dense chocolate cake is definitely for an adult crowd. If the sour cream icing is not to your taste, try the Brownie Fudge Cake with a more traditional chocolate frosting (see page 69).

CAKE
3/4 cup packed brown sugar
1/2 cup granulated sugar
1/2 cup unsweetened cocoa powder
1/3 cup vegetable oil
2 large eggs
1/2 cup water
2 tsp vanilla
1 1/4 cups all-purpose flour
1 1/2 tsp baking powder
1/2 tsp baking soda
1 cup low-fat sour cream
   (room temperature)

ICING
1 cup low-fat sour cream
1 1/4 cups icing sugar
3 tbsp unsweetened cocoa powder
1 1/2 oz semi-sweet chocolate
   or 3 tbsp semi-sweet chocolate
   chips

Preheat the oven to 350°F. Spray a 9-inch square cake pan with vegetable spray.

1. Make cake: In a large bowl and using a whisk or electric mixer, beat brown sugar, sugar, cocoa, oil, eggs, water, and vanilla.
2. In another bowl, stir together flour, baking powder, and baking soda. With a wooden spoon, stir the dry ingredients into the cocoa mixture in batches, alternating with the sour cream, just until combined. Pour the mixture into a prepared pan.
3. Bake in the centre of the oven for 20 to 25 minutes or until a tester comes out dry.
4. Let the pan cool on a wire rack.
5. Make icing: In a microwaveable bowl, heat the chocolate on high for 30 seconds. Stir the mixture until it is smooth. In a food processor, beat sour cream, icing sugar, cocoa, and melted chocolate together until the mixture is smooth. Pour over the top and sides of the cake.

black forest cake with italian meringue

From Germany's Black Forest, this chocolate cake is usually flavoured with kirsch, liqueur, decorated with sour cherries, and layered with whipped cream. My version is far lower in fat and calories.

CAKE
2 tsp instant coffee granules
1/4 cup hot water
3/4 cup granulated sugar
1/3 cup vegetable oil
1 large egg
1 large egg white
1 1/2 tsp vanilla
3/4 cup all-purpose flour

1/3 cup unsweetened cocoa
   powder
1 1/2 tsp baking powder
1/2 tsp baking soda
1/4 tsp salt
3/4 cup low-fat sour cream

ICING
3 large egg whites
3/4 cup granulated sugar
1/4 cup water
1/4 tsp cream of tartar
1/4 cup raspberry jam
1/4 cup dried cherries
1/2 oz semi-sweet chocolate,
   grated

MAKES 12 SERVINGS

NUTRITIONAL ANALYSIS
PER SERVING
Energy 253 calories
Protein 3.4 g
Fat, total 8.4 g
Fat, saturated 1.8 g
Carbohydrates 41 g
Fibre 1.1 g
Cholesterol 23 mg

Preheat the oven to 350°F. Spray two 8-inch round cake pans with vegetable spray.

1. Make cake: Dissolve instant coffee in hot water.
2. In a large bowl and using a whisk or electric mixer, beat cooled coffee, sugar, oil, egg, egg white, and vanilla.
3. In another bowl, stir together flour, cocoa, baking powder, baking soda, and salt. With a wooden spoon, stir the dry ingredients into the sugar mixture in batches, alternating with the sour cream, just until combined. Divide the mixture between the prepared pans.
4. Bake in the centre of the oven for 15 minutes or until a tester inserted in centre comes out with just a few crumbs clinging to it. Let the pans sit on a wire rack for 10 minutes. Remove the cakes from the pans and set them on racks to cool.
5. Make icing: In the top of a double boiler or in a glass or metal bowl that fits over top a saucepan of simmering water, combine egg whites, sugar, water, and cream of tartar. Place pan over medium-low heat. With an electric mixer, beat for 8 minutes or until mixture thickens and soft peaks form. Remove the pan from the heat; beat the mixture for 1 minute or until stiff peaks form.
6. Place one cake layer on a cake platter. On the stovetop or in the microwave, heat the jam; spread it over the cake layer. Sprinkle with dried cherries. Spread some icing over top. Place the second cake layer on top of the first and ice the top and sides. Sprinkle with chocolate.

NUTRITION WATCH
Whipped cream contains 35% MF, compared to this Italian meringue icing, which contains no fat at all. Once you've tried it, you may well choose the meringue as regular icing for all your cakes.

TIP
I like to use dried cherries because sour cherries are not easy to find and are often not pitted. By all means use sour cherries if they're available, and pit them.

coconut layer cake
with italian meringue icing

I used to avoid coconut desserts because coconut milk contains saturated fat. Now that light coconut milk, which is 75% reduced in fat, is available I even add it where it's not called for!

CAKE
1 cup granulated sugar
3/4 cup light coconut milk
1/3 cup vegetable oil
2 large eggs
1 1/2 tsp vanilla
1 1/4 cups all-purpose flour

1 1/2 tsp baking powder
1/4 tsp salt
5 tbsp toasted coconut
2 large egg whites
1/4 tsp cream of tartar
1/4 cup granulated sugar

ICING
3 large egg whites
3/4 cup granulated sugar
1/4 cup water
1/4 tsp cream of tartar

Preheat the oven to 350°F. Spray two 9-inch round cake pans with vegetable spray.

1. Make cake: In a large bowl and using a whisk or electric mixer, beat 1 cup sugar, coconut milk, oil, eggs, and vanilla.

2. In another bowl, stir together flour, baking powder, salt, and 2 tbsp toasted coconut. With a wooden spoon, stir the dry ingredients into the coconut milk mixture just until combined.

3. In a separate bowl, beat egg whites with cream of tartar until they are foamy. Gradually add 1/4 cup sugar, beating until stiff peaks form. Stir one quarter of egg whites into the cake batter. Gently fold in the remaining egg whites. Divide the mixture between the prepared pans.

4. Bake in the centre of the oven for approximately 15 minutes or until a tester inserted into the centre comes out dry. Let the pans cool on a wire rack.

5. Make icing: In the top of a double boiler or in a glass or metal bowl over top of a saucepan of simmering water, combine egg whites, sugar, water, and cream of tartar. Place over medium heat. With an electric mixer, beat for 6 to 8 minutes or until it is thickened and soft peaks form. Remove it from heat; beat for 1 minute or until stiff peaks form. Stir in 2 tbsp toasted coconut.

6. Place one cake layer on a cake platter. Spread some icing over top. Place the second cake layer on top of the first and ice the top and sides. Sprinkle with 1 tbsp toasted coconut.

orange layer cake
with cream cheese frosting

An orange cake with a creamy cheese-based icing, light and fluffy as a cloud. Orange juice concentrate gives this cake its intense orange flavour.

CAKE

1 cup granulated sugar

1/3 cup vegetable oil

2 large eggs

1/3 cup orange juice concentrate

1 tbsp finely grated orange rind

1 1/4 cups all-purpose flour

1 1/2 tsp baking powder

1 tsp baking soda

1 cup low-fat yogurt

ICING

1 1/4 cups smooth 5% ricotta
  cheese

2 1/2 oz light cream cheese, softened

3/4 cup granulated sugar

1 1/2 tbsp orange juice concentrate

2 tsp finely grated orange rind

Preheat the oven to 350°F. Spray two 9-inch round cake pans with vegetable spray.

1. Make cake: In a large bowl and using a whisk or electric mixer, beat sugar, oil, eggs, orange juice concentrate, and orange rind.

2. In another bowl, stir together flour, baking powder, and baking soda. With a wooden spoon, stir the dry ingredients into the sugar mixture in batches, alternating with the yogurt, just until combined. Divide the mixture between the prepared pans.

3. Bake in the centre of the oven for 15 to 20 minutes or until a tester comes out dry.

4. Let the pans cool on a wire rack.

5. Make icing: In a food processor, combine ricotta cheese, cream cheese, sugar, orange juice concentrate, and orange rind; purée until smooth. Transfer the mixture to a bowl and cover with plastic wrap. Chill until the cakes are fully cooled.

6. Place one cake layer on a cake platter. Spread some icing over top. Place the second cake layer on top of the first and ice the top and sides.

MAKES 14 SERVINGS

NUTRITIONAL ANALYSIS
PER SERVING
Energy 263 calories
Protein 6.2 g
Fat, total 8.5 g
Fat, saturated 2.4 g
Carbohydrates 40 g
Fibre 0.4 g
Cholesterol 41 mg

NUTRITION WATCH
Regular cake icing contains
mostly butter, lard, or vegetable shortening — 2 tbsp
of icing have 150 calories
and 8 g of fat. The icing for
this cake is made from
5% ricotta cheese and a
small amount of low-fat
cream cheese so the fat and
calorie content is very low.

TIP
When grating an orange or
lemon, be sure not to grate
the white pith under the skin.
It is bitter and will destroy
the taste of your dessert.

boston cream pie

A delicious dessert usually made with sponge layers and a filling of egg- and cream-based custard and whipping cream, the traditional version of this cake is very rich and filled with fat and calories. My version uses a combination of ricotta and cream cheese and orange to heighten the heavenly flavour.

CUSTARD
1/2 cup smooth 5% ricotta
   cheese
2 oz light cream cheese
1/3 cup granulated sugar
2 tbsp orange juice
   concentrate
2 tsp grated orange rind

CAKE
1 cup granulated sugar
1/4 cup vegetable oil
1 large egg
2 large egg whites
1 1/2 tsp vanilla
1 1/4 cups all-purpose flour
2 tsp baking powder
1/8 tsp salt
3/4 cup low-fat yogurt

GLAZE
3 tbsp semi-sweet
   chocolate chips
1 1/2 tbsp water

Preheat the oven to 350°F. Spray two 9-inch round cake pans with vegetable spray.

1. Make custard: In a food processor, combine ricotta, cream cheese, sugar, orange juice concentrate, and rind. Purée until the mixture is smooth. Chill while you prepare the cakes.

2. Make cake: In a large bowl and using a whisk or electric mixer, beat sugar, oil, egg, egg whites, and vanilla. In another bowl, stir together flour, baking powder, and salt. With a wooden spoon, stir the dry ingredients into the sugar mixture in batches, alternating with the yogurt, just until combined. Divide the mixture between the prepared pans.

3. Bake in the centre of the oven for 12 to 15 minutes or until a tester inserted in the centre comes out dry.

4. Let the pans cool on a wire rack.

5. Place one cake layer on a cake platter. Spread the custard over top. Place the second cake layer on top of the first.

6. Make glaze: In a microwave, melt the chocolate with water on high for 20 seconds or just until the chocolate begins to melt. Stir until it is smooth and pour over top in a marble design.

cheesecakes

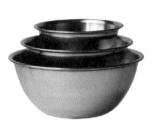

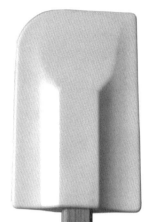

tips for divine light cheesecakes

1. Read the recipe carefully to make sure you have all the necessary ingredients or substitutions, preferably at room temperature. However, it's not necessary if you beat your ingredients thoroughly. Preheat your oven to the correct temperature.

2. Use a food processor with a metal blade for cheesecakes because ricotta or cottage cheese both have a grainy texture. A hand or electric beater does not always make a smooth batter.

3. Most recipes call for a 9-inch springform pan, which is a metal pan with a removable bottom. If you must use a different size, adjust the cooking time accordingly — for a smaller pan, add 10 minutes per inch, and for a larger pan, subtract 10 minutes per inch.

4. Ricotta cheese contains much less fat than regular cream cheese (between 5% and 10% MF, compared to cream cheese's 35% MF). Light cream cheese lends richness with less fat. You can substitute 2% MF cottage cheese for the ricotta cheese.

5. Egg whites give a light and fluffy texture. When beating them, always be sure that the bowl and beater are totally clean or they will not foam properly. If that happens, add 2 tsp lemon juice for every 2 egg whites. Pour the whites into the rest of the batter slowly in stages, folding just enough to incorporate them. Overfolding causes egg whites to lose their volume.

6. Don't worry about overmixing a cheesecake — keep processing the batter, scraping down the sides until the batter looks smooth and velvety.

7. I set my oven rack in the centre and always place the cheesecake pan on a jelly roll pan, since liquid from the crust can leak.

8. Cheesecakes are notorious for cracking. Cracks occur because the cake has released its moisture or steam too quickly, which can be caused by extreme temperatures. Place a pan of water on the bottom rack in the oven. Never open the oven door until the cheesecake is almost done. Do not place a cheesecake fresh out of the oven in a cool or drafty place. Run a butter knife around the sides of the pan, to release the tension. If all else fails, top the cheesecake with sliced fruit.

9. A cheesecake is done when the 2-inch diameter at the centre is slightly loose. If it bakes until it is firm in the centre, the cheesecake will be too dry. Remember — it will harden as it cools.

10. After the cheesecake is baked, let it cool to room temperature and then chill it for at least 2 hours. Cheesecake tastes best when it is thoroughly chilled.

11. You can freeze cheesecakes that do not contain whipped egg whites. Wrap the cake carefully in plastic wrap or foil and place it in a freezer bag for up to 3 months.

mango swirl cheesecake

I find cheesecakes with fruit to be luscious. In this version, puréed mango is swirled through the cheesecake. For some extra mango flavour, serve with Mango Coulis (see page 243).

PURÉE
Half ripe mango, peeled and pitted

CRUST
1 3/4 cups graham cracker crumbs
2 tbsp granulated sugar
3 tbsp water
1 tbsp liquid honey
1 tbsp vegetable oil

FILLING
2 cups 2% cottage cheese
4 oz light cream cheese, softened
1 cup granulated sugar
3/4 cup low-fat sour cream
1 large egg
2 large egg whites
1/4 cup all-purpose flour
2 tsp finely grated orange rind
1 1/2 tsp vanilla

Preheat the oven to 350°F. Spray a 9-inch springform pan with vegetable spray.

1. Make purée: In a food processor or blender, purée mango. Set it aside.
2. Make crust: In a bowl, stir together graham crumbs, sugar, water, honey, and oil until mixed. Pat mixture onto the bottom and side of a prepared pan.
3. Make filling: In the clean bowl of a food processor, combine cottage cheese, cream cheese, sugar, sour cream, egg, egg whites, flour, orange rind, and vanilla; purée until smooth. Pour the mixture into the crust. Dollop the puréed mango over top of the batter and use a butter knife to swirl it around.
4. Place a pan of hot water on the bottom rack of the oven. Bake the cheesecake in the centre of the oven for 55 to 60 minutes or until it is slightly loose at the centre.
5. Run a butter knife around the edge of the cake. Let the pan cool on a wire rack until it is room temperature. Chill.

MAKES 16 SERVINGS

NUTRITIONAL ANALYSIS
PER SERVING
Energy 198 calories
Protein 7 g
Fat, total 5.1 g
Fat, saturated 2.1 g
Carbohydrates 3.1 g
Fibre 0.6 g
Cholesterol 23 mg

NUTRITION WATCH
Mango is rich in vitamins A, C, and D, and in potassium and fibre. Fresh mangoes are available between May and September.

TIP
You can replace the cottage cheese with ricotta cheese for a creamier texture. Be sure to process it well to get rid of any lumps.

cranberry swirl cheesecake

MAKES 16 SERVINGS

NUTRITIONAL ANALYSIS
PER SERVING
Energy 187 calories
Protein 4.5 g
Fat, total 6.8 g
Fat, saturated 2.8 g
Carbohydrates 27 g
Fibre 0.4 g
Cholesterol 28 mg

NUTRITION WATCH
Ricotta is a good source of
calcium and now comes in
5% MF. I use it in place of
cream cheese, so I reduce
the amount of fat by as much
as half.

TIPS
Vanilla wafers come whole
in a box. To make crumbs,
place all the wafers in the
food processor and purée
until they are ground; then
you can measure them.

If you substitute graham
crackers, add 2 tbsp sugar.

For the ultimate flavour and texture, use canned, whole-berry cranberry sauce — not the jellied
version — for this colourful cake. When I tried whole cranberries, they fell to the bottom of the
pan and provided too tart a flavour.

PURÉE
1/2 cup canned whole-berry
   cranberry sauce

CRUST
2 cups vanilla wafer crumbs
1 tbsp vegetable oil
2 tbsp water

FILLING
1 1/2 cup smooth 5% ricotta cheese
3 oz light cream cheese, softened
2/3 cup low-fat sour cream
1 large egg
2 tsp vanilla
3/4 cup granulated sugar
3 tbsp all-purpose flour

Preheat the oven to 350°F. Spray a 9-inch springform pan with vegetable spray.

1. Make purée: In a food processor or blender, purée the cranberry sauce. Set it aside.
2. Make crust: In a bowl, stir together wafer crumbs, oil, and water until mixed. Pat the mixture
   onto the bottom and side of a prepared pan.
3. Make filling: In the clean bowl of a food processor, combine ricotta cheese, cream cheese, sour
   cream, egg, vanilla, sugar, and flour; purée until smooth. Pour the mixture into the crust. Dollop
   the puréed cranberry sauce over the batter and use a butter knife to swirl it around.
4. Place a pan of hot water on the bottom rack of the oven. Bake the cheesecake in the centre of
   the oven for 45 minutes or until it is slightly loose at the centre.
5. Run a butter knife around the edge of the cake. Let it cool on a wire rack until it is room
   temperature. Chill.

apricot swirl cheesecake

When dried fruit is rehydrated, it makes a wonderful purée. And dried apricots lend their intense flavour for this incredibly delicious cheesecake.

APRICOT SWIRL
3 oz (1/2 cup) chopped dried
  apricots
1 cup water
3 tbsp granulated sugar

CRUST
1 3/4 cup graham cracker
  crumbs

3 tbsp granulated sugar
1/4 cup water
1 tbsp vegetable oil

FILLING
2 cups 2% cottage cheese
4 oz light cream cheese,
  softened
1/2 cup low-fat sour cream

1 large egg
1 tsp vanilla
1 tsp finely grated lemon rind
1 tbsp lemon juice
3/4 cup granulated sugar
1/4 cup all-purpose flour
2 large egg whites
1/4 tsp cream of tartar
1/4 cup granulated sugar

Preheat the oven to 350°F. Spray a 9-inch springform pan with vegetable spray.

1. Make apricot swirl: In a small saucepan, combine apricots, water, and sugar. Bring the mixture to a boil. Reduce heat to medium-low and simmer for 12 to 15 minutes or until the apricots are tender. In a food processor or blender, purée the mixture until it is smooth. Set it aside.
2. Make crust: In a bowl, stir together graham crumbs, sugar, water, and oil until combined. Pat the mixture onto the bottom and side of a prepared pan.
3. Make filling: In the clean bowl of a food processor, combine cottage cheese, cream cheese, sour cream, egg, vanilla, lemon rind, lemon juice, 3/4 cup sugar, and flour; purée until smooth. Transfer the mixture to a large bowl and set it aside.
4. In another bowl, beat egg whites with cream of tartar until they are foamy. Gradually add 1/4 cup sugar, continuing to beat until stiff peaks form. Gently fold the egg mixture into the cheese mixture just until combined. Pour the mixture into the prepared crust. Dollop the puréed apricot over the batter and use a butter knife to swirl it around.
5. Place a pan of hot water on the bottom rack of the oven. Bake the cheesecake in the centre of the oven for 50 to 55 minutes or until it is slightly loose at the centre.
6. Run a butter knife around the edge of the cake. Let it cool on a wire rack until it is room temperature. Chill.

MAKES 16 SERVINGS

NUTRITIONAL ANALYSIS
PER SERVING
Energy 211 calories
Protein 7 g
Fat, total 4.8 g
Fat, saturated 1.9 g
Carbohydrates 35 g
Fibre 0.9 g
Cholesterol 2.2 mg

NUTRITION WATCH
Apricots are rich in vitamin A and are a valuable source of iron and calcium. They are a concentrated form of energy, so they make a great energizing snack any time.

TIPS
Ricotta can replace the cottage cheese for a creamier, denser cake.

Buy dried apricots in bulk and keep them in the freezer; you can use scissors to cut them into pieces.

coconut cream cheesecake

MAKES 16 SERVINGS

NUTRITIONAL ANALYSIS
PER SERVING
Energy 230 calories
Protein 6.2 g
Fat, total 9.5 g
Fat, saturated 4.7 g
Carbohydrates 30 g
Fibre 0.8 g
Cholesterol 28 mg

NUTRITION WATCH
Coconut is high in fat so use
it to highlight, not dominate,
a recipe. It is also high in
potassium.

TIPS
If ricotta is not available, use
2% cottage cheese and purée
it well to get rid of curds.

Toast the coconut in a skillet
over a high heat for 2 to 3
minutes until it is browned.

I would never have made this delicious cheesecake with regular coconut milk, which is laden with calories, fat, and cholesterol. But now that light coconut milk, which has 75% less fat, is available in my grocery store, I can indulge.

CRUST
2 1/4 cups vanilla wafer
   crumbs
2 tbsp granulated sugar
2 tbsp toasted coconut
1/4 cup water
1 tbsp vegetable oil

FILLING
2 cups smooth 5%
   ricotta cheese
4 oz light cream cheese,
   softened
3/4 cup light coconut milk
1 large egg
1 large egg white
2 tsp vanilla
3/4 cup granulated sugar
1/4 cup all-purpose flour

1/8 tsp salt
1/4 cup toasted coconut
2 large egg whites
1/4 tsp cream of tartar
2 tbsp granulated sugar

TOPPING
1 tbsp toasted coconut

Preheat the oven to 350°F. Spray a 9-inch springform pan with vegetable spray.

1. Make crust: In a bowl, stir together wafer crumbs, sugar, coconut, water, and oil until mixed. Pat the mixture onto the bottom and side of a prepared pan.
2. Make filling: In a food processor, combine ricotta cheese, cream cheese, coconut milk, egg, egg white, vanilla, sugar, flour, and salt; purée until smooth. Transfer the mixture to a large bowl. Stir in 1/4 cup coconut.
3. In another bowl, beat egg whites with cream of tartar until they are foamy. Gradually add 2 tbsp sugar, continuing to beat until stiff peaks form. Gently fold the egg mixture into the cheese mixture just until blended. Pour into the prepared crust.
4. Place a pan of hot water on the bottom rack of the oven. Bake the cheesecake in the centre of the oven for 55 to 60 minutes or until it is slightly loose at the centre.
5. Run a butter knife around the edge of the cake. Let it cool on a wire rack until it is room temperature. Chill.
6. Make topping: Garnish with 1 tbsp toasted coconut.

new york–style mocha cheesecake

The traditional New York cheesecake is dense, heavy, and oh so rich! Yes, it is delicious but it is also loaded with calories, fat, and cholesterol. Thanks to beaten egg whites, this mocha version is so light, you'll wake up feeling great. Serve it with a fruit coulis or chocolate sauce (see Sauces).

CRUST
1 cup chocolate wafer
   crumbs
3/4 cup graham cracker
   crumbs
3 tbsp granulated sugar
3 tbsp water
1 tbsp vegetable oil

FILLING
1 tbsp instant coffee granules
2 tbsp hot water
1 1/2 cups smooth 5%
   ricotta cheese
3 oz light cream cheese,
   softened
2 large eggs, separated
1 1/2 tsp vanilla
3/4 cup low-fat yogurt

1 cup granulated sugar
1/4 cup all-purpose flour
1/4 tsp cream of tartar
3 tbsp granulated sugar

CHOCOLATE SWIRL
1/4 cup semi-sweet chocolate
   chips
1 tbsp hot water

Preheat the oven to 350°F. Spray a 9-inch springform pan with vegetable spray.

1. Make crust: In a bowl, stir together wafer crumbs, graham crumbs, sugar, water, and oil until mixed. Pat the mixture onto the bottom and side of a prepared pan.
2. Make filling: Dissolve coffee in hot water. Place it in a food processor along with ricotta cheese, cream cheese, egg yolks, vanilla, yogurt, 1 cup sugar, and flour; purée until smooth. Transfer the mixture to a large bowl.
3. In another bowl, beat egg whites with cream of tartar until they are foamy. Gradually add 3 tbsp sugar, continuing to beat until stiff peaks form. Gently fold the egg mixture into the cheese mixture just until blended. Pour it into the prepared crust.
4. Make chocolate swirl: In a microwavable bowl, heat the chocolate chips with water on high for 40 seconds. Stir the mixture until it is smooth. Place dollops over top of the filling and use a butter knife to swirl it around.
5. Place a pan of hot water on the bottom rack of the oven. Bake the cheesecake in the centre of the oven for 55 to 60 minutes or until it is slightly loose at the centre.
6. Run a butter knife around the edge of the cake. Let it cool on a wire rack until it is room temperature. Chill.

MAKES 16 SERVINGS

NUTRITIONAL ANALYSIS
PER SERVING
Energy 218 calories
Protein 5.8 g
Fat, total 7 g
Fat, saturated 2.9 g
Carbohydrates 33 g
Fibre 0.6 g
Cholesterol 37 mg

NUTRITION WATCH
With the amount of cheese
and yogurt in this recipe, it
is a good source of calcium
and protein. Dessert can be
nutritious!

TIP
If you don't have instant
coffee on hand, use 2 tbsp
strong brewed coffee left
over from breakfast.

new york–style cheesecake with glazed strawberry topping

MAKES 16 SERVINGS

NUTRITIONAL ANALYSIS
PER SERVING
Energy 210 calories
Protein 5.7 g
Fat, total 6.6 g
Fat, saturated 2.8 g
Carbohydrates 32 g
Fibre 0.7 g
Cholesterol 40 mg

NUTRITION WATCH
Strawberries are an excellent source of vitamin C, and provide potassium and iron. They also play a role in cancer prevention.

TIPS
To make wafer crumbs, place whole wafers in the food processor and grind until they reach the desired consistency. Then measure out what you need.

You can always substitute graham crackers.

This is one of my favourite cheesecake recipes. It's light and airy yet tastes rich and satisfying. Serve this with Strawberry Coulis (see page 242).

CRUST
1 3/4 cups vanilla wafer
  crumbs
2 tbsp granulated sugar
2 tbsp water
1 tbsp margarine or butter

FILLING
1 1/2 cups smooth 5%
  ricotta cheese
1 cup low-fat yogurt
4 oz light cream cheese,
  softened
2 large eggs, separated
1 1/2 tsp vanilla
1 cup granulated sugar
1/4 cup all-purpose flour
1/8 tsp salt
1/4 tsp cream of tartar
2 tbsp granulated sugar

TOPPING
2 cups sliced strawberries
2 tbsp red currant jelly or
  apple jelly

Preheat the oven to 350°F. Spray a 9-inch springform pan with vegetable spray.

1. Make crust: In a bowl, stir together wafer crumbs, sugar, water, and margarine until mixed. Pat the mixture onto the bottom and side of a prepared pan.
2. Make filling: In a food processor, combine ricotta cheese, yogurt, cream cheese, egg yolks, vanilla, 1 cup sugar, flour, and salt; purée until smooth. Transfer the mixture to a large bowl.
3. In another bowl and using a whisk or electric beater, beat egg whites with cream of tartar until they are foamy. Gradually add 2 tbsp sugar, continuing to beat until stiff peaks form. Gently fold the mixture into the cheese mixture just until incorporated. Pour it into prepared crust.
4. Place a pan of hot water on the bottom rack of the oven. Bake the cheesecake in the centre of the oven for 55 to 60 minutes or until it is slightly loose at the centre.
5. Run a butter knife around the edge of the cake. Let it cool on a wire rack until it is room temperature.
6. Make topping: Arrange strawberries on top of the cheesecake. In a microwave or on the stovetop, heat the jelly until it is melted. Brush over the berries. Chill.

molasses ginger cheesecake

I love the flavour of gingerbread, whether it's in a cookie or cake. When combined in a cheesecake, it's exceptional.

CRUST

1 3/4 cups ladyfinger crumbs
2 tbsp granulated sugar
1/2 tsp ground cinnamon
1/4 cup water
1 tbsp liquid honey
1 tbsp vegetable oil

FILLING

2 cups smooth 5% ricotta cheese
3 oz light cream cheese
1 large egg
3/4 cup low-fat sour cream
1/3 cup molasses
2/3 cup packed brown sugar
1/3 cup granulated sugar
3 tbsp all-purpose flour
1 tsp ground cinnamon
1/4 tsp ground ginger
2 large egg whites
1/4 tsp cream of tartar
1/4 cup granulated sugar

Preheat the oven to 350°F. Spray a 9-inch springform pan with vegetable spray.

1. Make crust: In a bowl, stir together ladyfinger crumbs, sugar, cinnamon, water, honey, and oil until mixed. Pat the mixture onto the bottom and side of a prepared pan.
2. Make filling: In a food processor, combine ricotta cheese, cream cheese, egg, sour cream, molasses, brown sugar, 1/3 cup sugar, flour, cinnamon, and ginger; purée until smooth. Transfer the mixture to a large bowl.
3. In another bowl and using a whisk or electric beater, beat egg whites with cream of tartar until they are foamy. Gradually add 1/4 cup sugar, continuing to beat until stiff peaks form. Gently fold the egg mixture into the cheese just until mixed. Pour it into the prepared crust.
4. Place a pan of hot water on the bottom rack of the oven. Bake the cheesecake in the centre of the oven for 60 to 65 minutes or until it is slightly loose at the centre.
5. Run a butter knife around the edge of the cake. Let it cool on a wire rack until it is room temperature. Chill.

MAKES 16 SERVINGS

NUTRITIONAL ANALYSIS
PER SERVING
Energy 223 calories
Protein 6.6 g
Fat, total 6.3 g
Fat, saturated 3.2 g
Carbohydrates 35 g
Fibre 0.3 g
Cholesterol 69 mg

NUTRITION WATCH
Molasses is rich in iron, calcium, and phosphorus.

TIPS
Buy firm, Italian packaged ladyfingers and process them in a food processor until the crumbs are fine.

You can substitute vanilla wafer or graham cracker crumbs — add just enough water for the crumbs to come together, keeping in mind that ladyfinger crumbs need more moisture.

lemon curd cheesecake

MAKES 16 SERVINGS

NUTRITIONAL ANALYSIS
PER SERVING
Energy 239 calories
Protein 6.8 g
Fat, total 6.6 g
Fat, saturated 2.8 g
Carbohydrates 38 g
Fibre 0.5 g
Cholesterol 34 mg

NUTRITION WATCH
Lemons are an excellent
source of vitamin C, but they
start to lose their vitamin
power as soon as they are
squeezed.

TIPS
For the best flavour, use fresh
lemon juice. In fact, I use
bottled lemon juice only if a
recipe does not depend on
lemon for its flavour.

To get the most juice from a
lemon, roll it firmly on a flat
surface before you cut it,
or heat it gently in the
microwave for 30 seconds.

Lemon is one of my favourite flavours in baking. Instead of using ordinary lemon in the cheesecake, I thought a marbled lemon curd would be delicious. It is!

LEMON CURD
1/3 cup granulated sugar
1 tbsp cornstarch
2/3 cup water
1 tsp finely grated lemon rind
2 tbsp fresh lemon juice
1 large egg

CRUST
1 3/4 cups graham cracker
    crumbs
3 tbsp granulated sugar
1/4 cup water
1 tbsp vegetable oil

FILLING
2 cups smooth 5% ricotta cheese
4 oz light cream cheese,
    softened

1 large egg
1 large egg white
1/2 cup low-fat plain or
    lemon-flavoured yogurt
2 tsp finely grated lemon
    rind
1/4 cup fresh lemon juice
1 1/3 cups granulated
    sugar
1/4 cup all-purpose flour

Preheat the oven to 350°F. Spray a 9-inch springform pan with vegetable spray.

1. Make curd: In a small saucepan off the heat, combine sugar, cornstarch, water, rind, and juice until smooth. Cook the mixture over medium heat, whisking constantly, for 4 minutes or until it is thickened. Remove the saucepan from heat. In a bowl, beat egg. Whisk the lemon mixture into the egg. Return the mixture to the saucepan and cook over the lowest heat, stirring constantly, for 3 minutes or until it is smooth and thickened. Transfer it to a clean bowl. Place a piece of plastic wrap on the surface of the lemon. Chill while you mix the cheesecake.

2. Make crust: In a bowl, stir together graham crumbs, sugar, water, and oil until mixed. Pat the mixture onto the bottom and side of a prepared pan.

3. Make filling: In a food processor, combine ricotta cheese, cream cheese, egg, egg white, yogurt, lemon rind and juice, sugar, and flour; purée until smooth. Pour the mixture into the prepared crust. Dollop the lemon curd on top of the filling and use a butter knife to swirl it around.

4. Place a pan of hot water on the bottom rack of the oven. Bake the cheesecake in the centre of the oven for approximately 60 minutes or until it is slightly loose at the centre.

5. Run a butter knife around the edge of the cake. Let it cool on a wire rack until it is room temperature. Chill.

sour cream brownie cheesecake

This cake is sinfully delicious — a thick layer of brownie topped with a creamy cheesecake layer and a light sour cream layer make it irresistible to kids and adults alike.

BROWNIE LAYER
2/3 cup granulated sugar
1/4 cup vegetable oil
1 large egg
1 tsp vanilla
1/3 cup all-purpose flour
1/3 cup unsweetened cocoa
   powder
1 tsp baking powder
1/4 cup low-fat sour cream

CHEESECAKE LAYER
1 cup smooth 5% ricotta
   cheese
1/2 cup granulated sugar
1/3 cup light cream cheese
1/4 cup low-fat sour cream
1 large egg
2 tbsp all-purpose flour
1 tsp vanilla
2 tbsp semi-sweet chocolate
   chips

TOPPING
1 cup low-fat sour cream
2 tbsp granulated sugar
1 tsp vanilla
1 tbsp semi-sweet chocolate
   chips

Preheat the oven to 350°F. Spray a 8 1/2-inch springform pan with vegetable spray.

1. Make brownie layer: In a bowl, beat together sugar, oil, egg, and vanilla. In another bowl, stir together flour, cocoa, and baking powder. Stir the wet mixture into the dry mixture just until combined. Stir in the sour cream. Pour the mixture into a prepared pan.
2. Make cheesecake layer: In a food processor, combine ricotta cheese, sugar, cream cheese, sour cream, egg, flour, and vanilla; process until smooth. Stir in chocolate chips. Pour the mixture on top of the brownie layer.
3. Place a pan of hot water on the bottom rack of the oven. Bake the cheesecake in the centre of the oven for 40 minutes. The brownie layer may rise slightly around the edges.
4. Make topping: In a small bowl, stir together sour cream, sugar, and vanilla.
5. When the cake layers have cooked, pour the topping mixture carefully over top, smoothing it with the back of a spoon, and sprinkle chocolate chips over top. Bake 10 more minutes. Let the pan cool on a wire rack. Chill before serving.

NUTRITIONAL ANALYSIS
PER SERVING
Energy 225 calories
Protein 7 g
Fat, total 8 g
Fat, saturated 3 g
Carbohydrates 31 g
Fibre 1 g
Cholesterol 47 mg

NUTRITION WATCH
Cheesecakes are often forbidden if you're trying to reduce calorie and fat intake. Usually they contain high-fat cream cheese, which has 35% MF, and regular sour cream, which has 14% MF, as well as many eggs. But this recipe uses low-fat sour cream and ricotta cheese and light cream cheese to reduce calories and fat.

TIP
For a mocha-flavoured brownie, add 1 tsp powdered coffee to 1 tbsp hot water or add 1 tbsp strong brewed coffee, to taste.

bailey's irish cream cheesecake

MAKES 16 SERVINGS

NUTRITIONAL ANALYSIS
PER SERVING
Energy 277 calories
Protein 8 g
Fat, total 9.9 g
Fat, saturated 4.6 g
Carbohydrates 39 g
Fibre 1.5 g
Cholesterol 34 mg

NUTRITION WATCH
Low-fat cheese, yogurt,
and sour cream are excellent
sources of protein and
calcium, and are low in
calories, fat, and cholesterol.

TIP
Feel free to substitute a
liqueur of your choice.
Try a combination of coffee
and chocolate!

Coffee cream liqueurs add a subtle flavour to desserts. Bailey's Irish Cream combined with a chocolate creamy cheesecake is not just delicious, it is decadent. Serve with one of the chocolate or raspberry sauces in Sauces.

CRUST
2 1/4 cups chocolate wafer
    crumbs
3 tbsp water
1 tbsp vegetable oil

FILLING
2 cups smooth 5% ricotta
    cheese
3/4 cup low-fat yogurt
4 oz light cream cheese
1 large egg
1 large egg white
2 tbsp Bailey's Irish Cream or
    other coffee cream liqueur
2 tsp vanilla
1 1/4 cups granulated sugar

1/2 cup unsweetened
    cocoa powder
3 tbsp all-purpose flour

TOPPING
1 1/4 cups low-fat sour
    cream
2 tbsp granulated sugar
1 tbsp Bailey's Irish Cream
    or other coffee cream
    liqueur

Preheat the oven to 350°F. Spray a 9-inch springform pan with vegetable spray.

1. Make crust: In a bowl, stir together wafer crumbs, water, and oil until mixed. Pat mixture onto the bottom and side of a prepared pan.
2. Make filling: In a food processor, combine ricotta cheese, yogurt, cream cheese, egg, egg white, liqueur, vanilla, sugar, cocoa, and flour; purée until smooth. Pour the mixture into the prepared crust.
3. Place a pan of hot water on the bottom rack of the oven. Bake the cheesecake in the centre of the oven for 50 minutes. The cake will still be quite loose.
4. Make topping: In a bowl, stir together sour cream, sugar, and liqueur. Carefully pour a thin stream of this mixture over top of the hot cheesecake, smoothing it with a knife. Return the cake to the oven and bake for 10 minutes. The topping will be loose and will set as the cake cools.
5. Run a butter knife around the edge of the cake. Let it cool on a wire rack until it is room temperature. Chill.

peanut butter chocolate swirl cheesecake

Your little angels will leave the peanut butter and jam sandwiches behind after they try this version of cheesecake. What a combination! Serve with Chocolate Sauce (see page 240).

CRUST
1 3/4 cups chocolate wafer
  crumbs
1 tbsp liquid honey
1 tbsp vegetable oil
2 tbsp water

FILLING
2 cups smooth 5% ricotta
  cheese
3/4 cup low-fat sour cream
3 oz light cream cheese,
  softened
1 large egg
1/3 cup smooth peanut butter
2 tsp vanilla
2/3 cup granulated sugar

3 tbsp all-purpose flour
2 large egg whites
1/4 tsp cream of tartar
3 tbsp granulated sugar

CHOCOLATE SWIRL
1/4 cup semi-sweet
  chocolate chips
1 tbsp water

NUTRITIONAL ANALYSIS
PER SERVING
Energy 246 calories
Protein 7.7 g
Fat, total 11 g
Fat, saturated 4.1 g
Carbohydrates 29 g
Fibre 1 g
Cholesterol 29 mg

NUTRITION WATCH
Peanut butter is a great
source of protein when
combined with a grain, as
in bread — perfect for
children who don't consume
enough protein in their diet.
Although it's high in fat, it
contains monounsaturated
fat, which is healthy.

TIP
Always buy natural smooth
peanut butter. The commercial brands can have hydrogenated fat and added sugar.

Preheat the oven to 350°F. Spray a 9-inch springform pan with vegetable spray.

1. Make crust: In a bowl, stir together wafer crumbs, honey, oil, and water until mixed. Pat mixture onto the bottom and side of a prepared pan.

2. Make filling: In a food processor, combine ricotta, sour cream, cream cheese, egg, peanut butter, vanilla, 2/3 cup sugar, and flour; purée until smooth. Transfer the mixture to a large bowl.

3. In another bowl and using an electric beater, beat egg whites with cream of tartar until they are foamy. Gradually add 3 tbsp sugar, continuing to beat until stiff peaks form. Gently fold the egg mixture into the cheese mixture just until blended and pour into a prepared crust.

4. Make chocolate swirl: In a microwavable bowl, heat chocolate chips with water on high for 40 seconds. Stir the mixture until it is smooth. Dollop the chocolate over top of the batter and use a butter knife to swirl it around.

5. Place a pan of hot water on the bottom rack of the oven. Bake the cheesecake in the centre of the oven for 45 to 50 minutes or until it is slightly loose at the centre.

6. Run a butter knife around the edge of the cake. Let it cool on a wire rack until it is room temperature. Chill.

rocky mountain miniature chocolate cheesecakes

MAKES 12 SERVINGS

NUTRITIONAL ANALYSIS
PER SERVING
Energy 161 calories
Protein 6.2 g
Fat, total 6.2 g
Fat, saturated 3.8 g
Carbohydrates 20 g
Fibre 0.6 g
Cholesterol 36 mg

NUTRITION WATCH
Light cream cheese is 25%
reduced in fat, compared to
regular cream cheese. It's still
filled with fat and calories,
so use it sparingly. I use it to
highlight a dessert.

TIPS
If you only have large marshmallows, use scissors to cut
them into small pieces.

You can replace the ricotta
with 2% cottage cheese —
just be sure to process it well
for a smooth batter.

I find that individual cheesecakes are elegant to serve, especially these ones, which are almost mousse-like in texture. Serve it with Chocolate Sauce (see page 240).

1 3/4 cups smooth 5% ricotta cheese
3 oz light cream cheese, softened
1/2 cup low-fat sour cream
1 large egg
3/4 cup granulated sugar
3 tbsp unsweetened cocoa powder
1 1/2 tbsp all-purpose flour
1/3 cup miniature marshmallows
3 tbsp semi-sweet chocolate chips

Preheat the oven to 350°F. Line one 12-cup muffin tin with paper muffin liners.

1. In a food processor, combine ricotta cheese, cream cheese, sour cream, egg, sugar, cocoa, and flour; purée until smooth. Divide the mixture among the prepared muffin cups.
2. Set the muffin tin in a larger pan. Pour enough hot water into the pan to come halfway up the sides of the muffin cups.
3. Bake in the centre of the oven for 20 minutes. Sprinkle marshmallows and chocolate chips evenly over cheesecakes. Bake for 5 minutes longer or until marshmallows and chocolate chips begin to melt.
4. Remove the muffin tin from its water bath. Let the tin cool on a wire rack. Chill.

miniature raspberry swirl cheesecakes

These individual desserts are a wonderful way to indulge your guests. I love to serve them with fresh fruit and Raspberry Coulis (see page 242). When raspberries are in season, use a few to decorate each cake.

1 1/4 cups smooth 5% ricotta cheese
1 1/4 cups 2% MF cottage cheese
1/3 cup low-fat sour cream
1 large egg
2 tsp vanilla
1 cup granulated sugar
1/4 cup all-purpose flour
1/3 cup raspberry jam

Preheat the oven to 350°F. Line one 12-cup muffin tin with paper muffin liners.

1. In a food processor, combine ricotta cheese, cottage cheese, sour cream, egg, vanilla, sugar, and flour; purée until smooth. Divide the mixture among the prepared muffin cups. Place a dollop of raspberry jam in each muffin cup and use a butter knife to swirl it around gently.
2. Set the muffin tin in a larger pan. Pour enough hot water into the pan to come halfway up the sides of the muffin cups.
3. Bake in the centre of the oven for 20 to 25 minutes or just until the muffins are set.
4. Remove the muffin tin from its water bath. Let the tin cool on a wire rack. Chill.

MAKES 12 SERVINGS

NUTRITIONAL ANALYSIS
PER SERVING
Energy 171 calories
Protein 7.2 g
Fat, total 3.4 g
Fat, saturated 2 g
Carbohydrates 28 g
Fibre 0.6 g
Cholesterol 36 mg

NUTRITION WATCH
Use 2% cottage cheese, rather than 1%, for better flavour and texture. Because the recipe is divided into 12 cheesecakes, the calories and fat won't vary much.

TIP
Cottage cheese makes these cheesecakes light and fluffy. Process it well for a smooth batter, and be sure to place a large pan filled with water in the oven to prevent the cakes from falling and to keep them moist.

coffee cakes, crumb cakes, and pound cakes

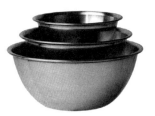

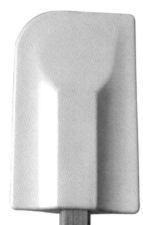

tips for divine light coffee cakes

1. Always preheat the oven and have all the ingredients on hand. It's better to have ingredients at room temperature.

2. Many of these coffee cakes are baked in 8-inch or 9-inch springform pans, which have a removable bottom. Spray the pan before using with vegetable spray.

3. Place the pan in the centre of the oven and check for doneness by inserting a toothpick or tester into the centre of the cake. The tester should come out dry and clean.

4. Cool the cake on a rack until it is room temperature.

5. Toppings add flavour and texture. Good topping ingredients to keep on hand are low-fat granola, quick-cooking rolled oats, and Grape-Nuts, which is a toasted wheat and barley low-fat cereal.

6. Some of the coffee cakes have puréed cooked dried fruit spooned over top for flavour and texture. Cook the fruit with the recommended amount of water, and mash or purée it until it is smooth. Just spoon it over top the batter and gently swirl it in. Do not mix it heavily or the fruit will sink to the bottom.

7. Italian meringue icing is a low-fat treat that requires beating the egg whites with sugar and water over a very low heat. This kills any bacteria in the egg whites and makes an icing that lasts much longer and is more stable than regular meringue toppings. Use it with any cake or muffin recipe. You can create a variety of icings by adding flavourings such as almond extract, orange juice concentrate, or cocoa.

cranberry sour cream coffee cake

Cranberries have a tartness that goes well with a sweet cake like this wonderful delight, especially combined with orange juice and a crunchy topping.

CAKE

1 tbsp finely grated orange rind
1/2 cup orange juice
1/2 cup low-fat sour cream
1/3 cup vegetable oil
1 large egg
2 large egg whites
2 tsp vanilla
1 cup granulated sugar
1 3/4 cups all-purpose flour
2 tsp baking powder
1 tsp baking soda
1 cup canned whole-berry
    cranberry sauce

TOPPING

1/4 cup Grape-Nuts cereal
3 tbsp packed brown sugar
3 tbsp all-purpose flour
2 tsp water
2 tsp vegetable oil

Preheat the oven to 350°F. Spray a 9-inch springform pan with vegetable spray.

1. Make cake: In a large bowl and using a whisk or electric mixer, beat orange rind and juice, sour cream, oil, egg, egg whites, vanilla, and sugar.

2. In another bowl, stir together flour, baking powder, and baking soda; with a wooden spoon, stir the flour mixture into the orange mixture just until it is combined. Pour the mixture into a prepared pan.

3. In a food processor, purée the cranberry sauce. Dollop it over the batter and use a butter knife to swirl it around gently.

4. Make topping: In a small bowl, stir together cereal, brown sugar, flour, water, and oil just until crumbly. Scatter the topping over the cake batter.

5. Place the pan in the centre of the oven and bake for 55 to 60 minutes or until a tester inserted in the centre of the cake comes out clean. Let the cake cool on a wire rack.

MAKES 16 SERVINGS

NUTRITIONAL ANALYSIS
PER SERVING
Energy 215 calories
Protein 2.9 g
Fat, total 6.1 g
Fat, saturated 0.9 g
Carbohydrates 37 g
Fibre 0.9 g
Cholesterol 16 mg

NUTRITION WATCH
Cranberries are a very good source of vitamin C. Dried cranberries make a great mid-day snack — their nutrients and calories are concentrated, and supply a quick energy source.

TIP
Canned cranberry sauce made with whole berries gives a better texture to the cake than whole cranberries on their own. Be careful not to buy jellied cranberry sauce.

orange apple sour cream coffee cake

Coffee cakes are a simple delicious cake to have any time of day, but this one puts coffee cakes in a different league completely. I like to serve it when I'm entertaining.

TOPPING
1/3 cup packed brown sugar
3 tbsp chopped pecans
1 1/2 tbsp all-purpose flour
2 tsp margarine or butter
1/2 tsp ground cinnamon

FILLING
2 cups peeled, chopped apples
1/2 cup raisins
1 tbsp granulated sugar
1 tsp ground cinnamon

CAKE
2/3 cup packed brown sugar
1/2 cup granulated sugar
1/3 cup vegetable oil
2 large eggs
1 tbsp grated orange rind
2 tsp vanilla
1 2/3 cups all-purpose flour
2 tsp baking powder
1 tsp baking soda
1/2 cup orange juice
1/2 cup low-fat sour cream

Preheat the oven to 350°F. Spray a 10-inch springform pan with vegetable spray.

1. Make topping: In a small bowl, combine brown sugar, pecans, flour, margarine, and cinnamon until crumbly. Set it aside.
2. Make filling: In a bowl, mix together apples, raisins, sugar, and cinnamon. Set it aside.
3. Make cake: In a large bowl and using a whisk or electric mixer, beat together brown sugar, granulated sugar, and oil. Add eggs one at a time, beating well after each. Mix in orange rind and vanilla.
4. In a separate bowl, stir together flour, baking powder, and baking soda. In another bowl, stir together orange juice and sour cream. Add the flour mixture and sour cream mixture in batches, alternating with the beaten sugar mixture, mixing just until it is all blended. Spoon half of the batter into a prepared pan. Top with half the apple mixture. Spoon the remaining batter into the pan. Top with the remaining apple mixture; sprinkle with topping.
5. Place the pan in the centre of the oven and bake for 45 to 50 minutes or until a tester inserted in the centre comes out clean. Let the pan cool on a wire rack.

raspberry coffee cake with granola topping

Tart raspberries go so well with the granola topping and sweet coffee cake.

TOPPING
1/3 cup packed brown sugar
1/4 cup low-fat granola
1/4 cup all-purpose flour
2 tsp water
2 tsp vegetable oil

CAKE
1 1/4 cups granulated sugar
1/3 cup vegetable oil
2 large eggs
1 1/2 tsp vanilla
1 1/3 cups all-purpose flour
1 1/2 tsp baking powder
1 tsp baking soda
1/8 tsp salt
3/4 cup low-fat yogurt
2 cups raspberries, fresh or
   thawed and drained
2 tsp all-purpose flour

Preheat the oven to 350°F. Spray a 9-inch square cake pan with vegetable spray.

1. Make topping: In a small bowl, mix together brown sugar, granola, flour, water, and oil until crumbly.
2. Make cake: In a large bowl and using a whisk or electric mixer, beat sugar, oil, eggs, and vanilla.
3. In another bowl, stir together 1 1/3 cups flour, baking powder, baking soda, and salt. With a wooden spoon, stir the dry ingredients into the sugar mixture in batches, alternating with the yogurt, making two additions of dry and one of wet, just until the mixture is combined.
4. Toss raspberries with 2 tsp flour and fold them into the batter. Pour the mixture into a prepared pan. Sprinkle with topping.
5. Place the pan in the centre of the oven and bake for 40 to 45 minutes or until a tester inserted in the centre comes out clean. Bake an extra 5 to 10 minutes if you are using frozen berries.
6. Let the pan cool on a wire rack.

MAKES 16 SERVINGS

NUTRITIONAL ANALYSIS
PER SERVING
Energy 204 calories
Protein 3 g
Fat, total 6.2 g
Fat, saturated 0.7 g
Carbohydrates 34 g
Fibre 1.5 g
Cholesterol 27 mg

NUTRITION WATCH
Be sure to buy low-fat granola (any flavour is fine), because regular granola is loaded with fat, calories, and cholesterol. Raspberries contain iron, potassium, and vitamins A and C.

TIPS
This recipe works well with either fresh or frozen raspberries. If you are using frozen berries, measure them before defrosting and then drain them.

orange marmalade coffee cake

Marmalade has a distinct tartness that goes well with this coffee cake and crunchy oatmeal topping. Serve it with Mango Coulis (see page 243).

MAKES 16 SERVINGS

NUTRITIONAL ANALYSIS
PER SERVING
Energy 217 calories
Protein 3.2 g
Fat, total 5.8 g
Fat, saturated 0.6 g
Carbohydrates 38 g
Fibre 0.7 g
Cholesterol 14 mg

NUTRITION WATCH
Despite its name, buttermilk
contains no butter — it is
just low-fat milk with added
bacteria to give it a slightly
thickened texture and tangy
flavour. It's great to use in
low-fat cooking.

TIPS
You can use apricot or peach
jam instead of marmalade.

You can also substitute low-
fat yogurt for buttermilk or
make your own buttermilk by
adding 1 tbsp lemon juice to
1 cup low-fat milk, and letting
it sit for 5 minutes.

CAKE
3/4 cup granulated sugar
2 tsp finely grated orange rind
1/2 cup orange juice
1/3 cup vegetable oil
1 large egg
2 large egg whites
1 tsp vanilla
1 3/4 cups all-purpose flour
1 1/2 tsp baking powder
1/2 tsp baking soda
3/4 cup buttermilk
2/3 cup marmalade

TOPPING
1/3 cup packed brown sugar
1/3 cup quick-cooking oats
1/4 cup all-purpose flour
1/2 tsp ground cinnamon
1 tbsp water
2 tsp vegetable oil

Preheat the oven to 350°F. Spray a 9-inch springform pan with vegetable spray.

1. Make cake: In a large bowl and using a whisk or electric mixer, beat sugar, orange rind and juice, oil, egg, egg whites, and vanilla.
2. In another bowl, stir together flour, baking powder, and baking soda. With a wooden spoon, stir the dry ingredients into the sugar mixture in batches, alternating with the buttermilk, making two additions of dry and one of wet, and stirring just until the mixture is combined. Pour it into a prepared pan.
3. Melt marmalade in a microwave or on the stove. Dot over the batter and gently swirl it around.
4. Make topping: In a small bowl, stir together brown sugar, oats, flour, cinnamon, water, and oil until crumbly. Sprinkle the mixture over the batter.
5. Place the pan in the centre of the oven and bake for 45 to 50 minutes or until a tester comes out dry.
6. Let cool on a wire rack.

upside-down apple and cranberry coffee cake

Upside-down cakes are attractive to serve. This one, dotted with dried cranberries, makes a very festive dessert.

TOPPING
1/4 cup corn syrup
3/4 cup packed brown sugar
1 tbsp margarine or butter
1/2 tsp ground cinnamon
1/4 cup thinly sliced, peeled apples
1/4 cup dried cranberries

CAKE
3/4 cup granulated sugar
1/3 cup unsweetened applesauce
1/4 cup vegetable oil
1 large egg
2 large egg whites
2 tsp vanilla
1 tsp ground cinnamon
1 1/4 cups all-purpose flour
1/2 tsp baking powder
1/2 cup low-fat yogurt

Preheat the oven to 350°F. Spray a 9-inch square cake pan with vegetable spray.

1. Make topping: In the cake pan, stir together corn syrup, brown sugar, margarine, and cinnamon. Place in the oven for 3 minutes or until the mixture is melted. Stir. The mixture will be sticky.
2. Place apples and cranberries on top.
3. Make cake: In a large bowl and using a whisk or electric mixer, combine sugar, applesauce, oil, egg, egg whites, vanilla, and cinnamon. In another bowl, stir together flour and baking powder. Stir the dry ingredients into the applesauce mixture in batches, alternating with the yogurt, making two additions of dry and one of wet, and stir just until the mixture is combined. Spread it over the fruit in the pan.
4. Place the pan in the centre of the oven and bake for 25 to 35 minutes or until a tester comes out dry.
5. Let cool on a wire rack for 20 minutes, then turn out on a large platter.

MAKES 16 SERVINGS

NUTRITIONAL ANALYSIS PER SERVING
Energy 192 calories
Protein 2.3 g
Fat, total 4.7 g
Fat, saturated 0.6 g
Carbohydrates 35 g
Fibre 0.8 g
Cholesterol 14 mg

NUTRITION WATCH
Between the apples and cranberries, you get vitamins A and C and a good source of fibre and carbohydrates with this cake.

TIP
Feel free to use other dried fruits such as dried cherries, raisins, chopped apricots, or dates.

prune-swirled coffee cake

MAKES 16 SERVINGS

NUTRITIONAL ANALYSIS
PER SERVING

Energy 175 calories

Protein 2.4 g

Fat, total 5.7 g

Fat, saturated 0.9 g

Carbohydrates 28 g

Fibre 0.7 g

Cholesterol 17 mg

NUTRITION WATCH

Prunes provide high energy
and fibre, and when they're
puréed they make a fabulous
no-fat substitute in baking,
giving moisture and texture.

TIPS

I buy dried fruits, such as
prunes, in a bulk food store
and keep large bags in the
freezer, so I never run out.

The sour cream can be
replaced with low-fat yogurt
with 1% MF or less.

I find that the combination of prunes and coffee produce a great-tasting coffee cake. I love a slice in the morning with a cup of coffee or, actually, any time of day.

PRUNE SWIRL

3 oz (1/2 cup) pitted prunes,
  chopped

2/3 cup water

2 tbsp granulated sugar

CAKE

2 tbsp instant coffee granules

1/3 cup hot water

1 cup granulated sugar

1/3 cup vegetable oil

1 large egg

1 large egg white

1 tsp vanilla

1 1/2 cups all-purpose flour

1 1/2 tsp baking powder

1/2 tsp baking soda

3/4 cup low-fat sour cream

Preheat the oven to 350°F. Spray a 8-inch square cake pan with vegetable spray.

1. Make prune swirl: In a small saucepan, combine prunes, water, and sugar. Bring the mixture to a boil; reduce the heat to simmer and cook for 10 minutes. In a food processor or blender, purée.
2. Make cake: Dissolve the instant coffee in hot water.
3. In a large bowl and using a whisk or electric mixer, beat sugar, oil, egg, egg white, vanilla, and coffee. In another bowl, stir together flour, baking powder, and baking soda. With a wooden spoon, stir the dry ingredients into the sugar mixture in batches, alternating with the sour cream, making two additions of dry and one of wet, and stirring just until the mixture is combined. Set aside 1/2 cup batter; pour the remaining batter into a prepared pan.
4. In a small bowl, stir together the prune purée and reserved batter. Dot over the batter in the pan and use a butter knife to swirl it around gently.
5. Place the pan in the centre of the oven and bake for 45 minutes or until a tester inserted in the centre comes out clean.
6. Let cool on a wire rack.

date oatmeal coffee cake

If you love date squares, you'll love this coffee cake. It's so moist, with a satisfying crunchy oatmeal topping.

CAKE
6 oz (1 1/4 cups) pitted dates, chopped
1 1/4 cups water
1 cup granulated sugar
2 large eggs
2 tsp vanilla
1 cup buttermilk
1/3 cup vegetable oil
1 1/3 cups all-purpose flour
1 1/2 tsp baking powder
1 tsp ground cinnamon
1/2 tsp baking soda

TOPPING
1/2 cup packed brown sugar
1/2 cup quick-cooking oats
1/4 cup all-purpose flour
1/2 tsp ground cinnamon
1 tbsp melted margarine or butter
1 tbsp water

Preheat the oven to 350°F. Spray a 9-inch springform pan with vegetable spray.

1. In a saucepan, combine dates and water. Bring the liquid to a boil; reduce the heat to medium and simmer uncovered for 5 to 8 minutes, stirring occasionally. Remove from heat. Mash. Let it cool while you prepare the topping and cake.
2. Make topping: In a small bowl, stir together brown sugar, oats, flour, cinnamon, margarine, and water until crumbly.
3. In a large bowl and using a whisk or electric mixer, beat sugar, eggs, vanilla, buttermilk, and oil. In another bowl, stir together flour, baking powder, cinnamon, and baking soda. Pour the wet ingredients over the dry ingredients; with a wooden spoon, stir the mixture just until it is combined. Pour it into a prepared pan. Dot the cooled date mixture on top. Sprinkle with topping.
4. Place the pan in the centre of the oven and bake for 50 to 55 minutes or until a tester inserted in the centre comes out clean.
5. Let cool on a wire rack.

MAKES 16 SERVINGS

NUTRITIONAL ANALYSIS
PER SERVING
Energy 226 calories
Protein 3.2 g
Fat, total 6.3 g
Fat, saturated 0.8 g
Carbohydrates 39 g
Fibre 1.5 g
Cholesterol 27 mg

NUTRITION WATCH
Dates are a good source of protein and iron. When they are cooked and puréed they can replace up to 75% of the fat in a baked dessert. For every cup of fat in a recipe, substitute 3/4 cup fruit purée, which equals 25% fat.

TIPS
As with all dried fruit, I buy pitted dates in bulk and keep them in the freezer. Use scissors to cut them into pieces.

Make your own buttermilk: add 1 tbsp lemon juice to 1 cup milk and let sit for 5 minutes.

mocha coffee cake

MAKES 16 SERVINGS

NUTRITIONAL ANALYSIS
PER SERVING
Energy 205 calories
Protein 2.7 g
Fat, total 6.5 g
Fat, saturated 1.5 g
Carbohydrates 34 g
Fibre 1.1 g
Cholesterol 17 mg

NUTRITION WATCH
The calories, fat, and
cholesterol are reduced in
this recipe by using mostly
cocoa instead of chocolate.
Cocoa has only 3 g of fat per
ounce, compared to 9 g of
fat in chocolate. With this
kind of saving, I can add a
few chocolate chips to the
topping.

TIPS
If you don't have brewed
coffee on hand, mix 1 tsp
instant coffee with 1/3 cup
hot water.

Substitute sour cream with
low-fat yogurt.

What can go wrong when you mix coffee with chocolate? I love a slice of this celestial cake with a cappuccino in the afternoon, especially when served with Crème Anglaise (see page 239) or Vanilla Cream (see page 241).

TOPPING
1/2 cup packed brown sugar
3 tbsp semi-sweet chocolate chips
4 tsp unsweetened cocoa powder

CAKE
1 1/4 cups granulated sugar
1/3 cup vegetable oil
1/3 cup brewed strong coffee
1 large egg
2 large egg whites
1 tsp vanilla
1 1/4 cups all-purpose flour
1/3 cup unsweetened cocoa powder
1 1/2 tsp baking powder
1/2 tsp baking soda
2/3 cup low-fat sour cream

Preheat the oven to 350°F. Spray a 9-inch square cake pan with vegetable spray.

1. Make topping: In a small bowl, stir together brown sugar, chocolate chips, and cocoa.
2. Make cake: In a large bowl and using whisk or electric mixer, beat sugar, oil, coffee, egg, egg whites, and vanilla.
3. In another bowl, stir together flour, cocoa, baking powder, and baking soda. With a wooden spoon, stir the dry ingredients into the coffee mixture in batches, alternating with the sour cream, making two additions of dry and one of wet, and stirring just until the mixture is combined. Pour it into a prepared pan. Sprinkle with topping.
4. Place the pan in the centre of the oven and bake for 30 to 35 minutes or until a tester inserted in the centre comes out clean.
5. Let cool on a wire rack.

cream cheese–filled coffee cake

This is one of my favourite coffee cakes. The combination of a light cream cheese layer and strawberry jam is incredible. Try serving it with Raspberry Coulis (see page 242).

FILLING
3/4 cup smooth 5% ricotta cheese
2 oz light cream cheese, softened
1 large egg yolk
1/4 cup granulated sugar
2 tsp all-purpose flour
1 tsp vanilla

TOPPING
1/3 cup Grape-Nuts cereal
3 tbsp all-purpose flour
3 tbsp packed brown sugar
1/4 tsp ground cinnamon
2 tsp vegetable oil
2 tsp water

CAKE
3/4 cup granulated sugar
3 tbsp vegetable oil
1 large egg
1 large egg white
2 tsp vanilla
1 cup all-purpose flour
1 1/2 tsp baking powder
1/2 tsp ground cinnamon
3/4 cup light sour cream
1/3 cup strawberry jam

Preheat the oven to 350°F. Spray a 8 1/2-inch springform pan with vegetable spray.

1. Make filling: In a food processor, combine ricotta cheese, cream cheese, egg yolk, sugar, flour, and vanilla; purée the mixture until it is smooth.
2. Make topping: In a small bowl, stir together cereal, flour, brown sugar, cinnamon, oil, and water until crumbly.
3. Make cake: In a large bowl and using a whisk or electric mixer, beat sugar, oil, egg, egg white, and vanilla. In another bowl, stir together flour, baking powder, and cinnamon. With a wooden spoon, stir the dry ingredients into the sugar mixture in batches, alternating with the sour cream, making two additions of dry and one of wet, and stirring the mixture just until it is combined. Pour it into a prepared pan.
4. Melt jam in a microwave or on the stovetop. Spread it over the cake batter. Pour the filling over top, spreading it to cover the batter. Sprinkle with the topping.
5. Place the pan in the centre of the oven and bake for 55 to 60 minutes or until a tester inserted in the centre comes out clean.
6. Let cool on a wire rack.

MAKES 16 SERVINGS

NUTRITIONAL ANALYSIS PER SERVING
Energy 196 calories
Protein 4.1 g
Fat, total 6.2 g
Fat, saturated 2 g
Carbohydrates 31 g
Fibre 0.5 g
Cholesterol 36 mg

NUTRITION WATCH
Grape-Nuts, a wheat and toasted barley cereal that makes a nutritious breakfast, gives a crunchy nutlike texture to desserts, without adding excess fat or calories.

TIPS
Substitute raspberry jam for strawberry.

Low-fat cottage cheese can replace ricotta cheese, but process it well until the mixture is free of lumps.

chocolate chip crumb cake

MAKES 16 SERVINGS

NUTRITIONAL ANALYSIS
PER SERVING
Energy 226 calories
Protein 5 g
Fat, total 7 g
Fat, saturated 4 g
Carbohydrates 36 g
Fibre 2 g
Cholesterol 42 mg

NUTRITION WATCH
Adapted from a recipe from
the Silver Palate bakery in
New York City. By using cocoa
and low-fat ricotta and
yogurt, I reduced the amount
of fat and calories for a
version that won't clog your
arteries so quickly! Even
though chocolate is higher in
fat and cholesterol than
cocoa, 1/2 cup spread over
16 slices is acceptable.
Here's proof you don't have
to eliminate chocolate when
you eat light!

TIP
A 9-inch springform pan can
be used instead of a Bundt
pan — check the cake at
30 to 40 minutes to see if it
needs to cook a few minutes
longer.

If I had to rate my number-one dessert of all time, this crumb cake would be it. I created it for *Enlightened Home Cooking,* and even today, I whip it up all the time. My children can now bake it blindfolded!

CAKE
8 oz smooth 5% ricotta cheese
1/3 cup margarine or butter
1 1/4 cups granulated sugar
2 large eggs
2 tsp vanilla
1 1/2 cups all-purpose flour
2 tsp baking powder
1/2 tsp baking soda
3/4 cup low-fat yogurt
1/2 cup semi-sweet chocolate
  chips

FILLING
1/2 cup packed brown sugar
4 tsp unsweetened cocoa
  powder
1/2 tsp ground cinnamon

Preheat the oven to 350°F. Spray a 9-inch Bundt pan with vegetable spray.

1. Make cake: In a large bowl or food processor, beat together ricotta cheese, margarine, and sugar, mixing well. Add the eggs and vanilla, mixing well.
2. Combine flour, baking powder, and baking soda; add the dry ingredients to the bowl in batches, alternating with the yogurt, mixing just until everything is incorporated. Stir in the chocolate chips. Pour half the batter into a prepared pan.
3. Make filling: Combine brown sugar, cocoa, and cinnamon in a small bowl. Sprinkle half over the batter in the pan. Add the remaining batter and top with the remaining filling.
4. Place the pan in the centre of the oven and bake for 35 to 40 minutes or until a tester inserted in the centre comes out dry.
5. Let the pan cool on a wire rack. After it has cooled, sprinkle with icing sugar, if desired.

white chocolate chip crumb cake

In my *Enlightened Home Cooking* cookbook, my favourite cake was the Chocolate Chip Crumb Cake. I adapted it to an all-chocolate version, dotted with white chocolate chips. It's so good!

CAKE
1 1/3 cups granulated sugar
1/3 cup unsweetened cocoa
   powder
1 cup smooth 5% ricotta cheese
1 large egg
2 large egg whites
1/3 cup vegetable oil
1 tsp vanilla
1 1/4 cups all-purpose flour
2/3 cup low-fat yogurt
1/3 cup white chocolate chips
2 tsp baking powder
1/2 tsp baking soda

CRUMB FILLING
1/2 cup packed brown sugar
4 tsp unsweetened cocoa
   powder

Preheat the oven to 350°F. Spray a 9-inch Bundt pan with vegetable spray.

1. Make cake: In a food processor, combine sugar, cocoa, ricotta cheese, egg, egg whites, oil, and vanilla; purée the mixture until it is smooth. Transfer it to a large bowl.
2. In another bowl, stir together flour, chips, baking powder, and baking soda. With a wooden spoon, stir the dry ingredients along with the yogurt into the sugar mixture just until everything is combined.
3. Make crumb filling: In a small bowl, stir together the brown sugar and cocoa.
4. Pour half of the batter into a prepared pan. Sprinkle with half of the crumb mixture. Pour the rest of the batter into the pan and sprinkle with the remaining crumb mixture.
5. Place the pan in the centre of the oven and bake for 35 to 40 minutes or until a tester comes out dry.
6. Let pan cool on a wire rack.

MAKES 16 SERVINGS

NUTRITIONAL ANALYSIS
PER SERVING
Energy 225 calories
Protein 4.2 g
Fat, total 7.6 g
Fat, saturated 2.1 g
Carbohydrates 35 g
Fibre 1 g
Cholesterol 19 mg

NUTRITION WATCH
Traditionally, a coffee cake like this one would be filled with much more fat, eggs, chocolate, and sour cream. By using ricotta cheese and cocoa, the amount of fat and calories is greatly reduced.

TIPS
I like to use a food processor with ricotta cheese so I can make the batter as smooth as possible.

If the cheese seems very dry, add 2 tbsp of milk to make it softer and smoother.

white and dark marble pound cake

The taste and texture of this pound cake are heavenly. By removing a small amount of the batter and mixing it with the cocoa mixture, you produce a beautiful marbled texture and appearance.

CAKE
1 1/4 cups granulated sugar
2 oz light cream cheese, softened
1/4 cup vegetable oil
1 large egg
1 large egg white
1 tbsp vanilla
2/3 cup low-fat yogurt
1 1/3 cups all-purpose flour
2 tsp baking powder

MARBLE
2 tbsp granulated sugar
4 tsp unsweetened cocoa powder
4 tsp water

TOPPING (OPTIONAL)
2 1/2 tbsp packed brown sugar
1/2 tsp unsweetened cocoa powder
2 tbsp semi-sweet chocolate chips

Preheat the oven to 350°F. Spray a 9-inch × 5-inch loaf pan with vegetable spray.

1. Make cake: In a large bowl and using a whisk or electric mixer, beat sugar, cream cheese, oil, egg, egg white, vanilla, and yogurt until the mixture is smooth.
2. In another bowl, stir together flour and baking powder. With a wooden spoon, stir the dry ingredients into the cream cheese mixture just until everything is combined. Remove 1/3 cup of the batter and set it aside. Pour the remaining batter into a prepared pan.
3. Make marble: In a small bowl, stir together reserved batter, sugar, cocoa, and water. Pour the mixture over top of the batter in the pan. Using a butter knife, swirl dark batter through light batter for a marbled effect.
4. Make topping: If desired, stir together brown sugar, cocoa, and chocolate chips. Sprinkle the mixture over the batter.
5. Place the pan in the centre of the oven and bake for 40 to 45 minutes or until a tester comes out dry.
6. Let the pan cool on a wire rack.

banana chocolate chip pound cake with streusel topping

This banana cake beats all the others. It is moist from the bananas and yogurt, and it has a delicious crunchy topping, with a few chocolate chips thrown in.

CAKE

3/4 cup granulated sugar

1 ripe (1/2 cup) large banana, mashed

1/4 cup vegetable oil

1 large egg

1 large egg white

2 tsp vanilla

1 cup low-fat yogurt

1 2/3 cups all-purpose flour

1 1/2 tsp baking powder

1/2 tsp baking soda

1/3 cup semi-sweet chocolate chips

TOPPING

1/3 cup Grape-Nuts cereal

1/4 cup packed brown sugar

1 tbsp all-purpose flour

1 1/2 tsp vegetable oil

1 tsp water

Preheat the oven to 350°F. Spray a 9-inch × 5-inch loaf pan with vegetable spray.

1. Make cake: In a large bowl and using a whisk or electric mixer, combine sugar, banana, oil, egg, egg white, vanilla, and yogurt.
2. In another bowl, stir together flour, baking powder, baking soda, and chocolate chips. With a wooden spoon, stir the dry ingredients into the banana mixture just until everything is combined. Pour the mixture into a prepared pan.
3. Make topping: In a bowl, stir together cereal, brown sugar, flour, oil, and water until combined. Sprinkle topping evenly over top.
4. Place the pan in the centre of the oven and bake for 40 to 45 minutes or until a tester comes out dry.
5. Let the pan cool on a wire rack.

MAKES 16 HALF SLICES

NUTRITIONAL ANALYSIS PER SERVING

Energy 194 calories

Protein 3 g

Fat, total 6.4 g

Fat, saturated 1.8 g

Carbohydrates 31 g

Fibre 1 g

Cholesterol 18 mg

NUTRITION WATCH

Grape-Nuts is a low-fat breakfast cereal made from toasted wheat and barley. Its nutty texture is delicious not only for breakfast, but also for use in baking without adding excess fat or calories.

TIP

For best results, use the ripest bananas you can find. In fact, keep overripe bananas in the freezer so they're handy for baking — just defrost and mash them. The intensity of the flavour is superb.

orange upside-down cake

NUTRITIONAL ANALYSIS
PER SERVING
Energy 184 calories
Protein 2.5 g
Fat, total 4.7 g
Fat, saturated 0.6 g
Carbohydrates 33 g
Fibre 0.8 g
Cholesterol 14 mg

NUTRITION WATCH

Oranges are an excellent source of vitamin C. But after being squeezed they begin losing some of their nutritional benefit.

TIP

Be sure to use sweet oranges or the cake will be bitter — taste them before you use them!

This cake looks so beautiful with the oranges caramelized on top. The cake beneath is moist and delicious.

2/3 cup packed brown sugar
1/4 cup corn syrup
1 tbsp margarine or butter
2 navel oranges
2/3 cup granulated sugar
Finely grated rind of 1 orange
1/2 cup low-fat yogurt
1/3 cup fresh orange juice
1/4 cup vegetable oil
1 large egg
2 large egg whites
1 1/3 cups all-purpose flour
1 1/2 tsp baking powder
1/8 tsp salt

Preheat the oven to 350°F. Spray a 9-inch square cake pan with vegetable spray.

1. In a prepared pan, stir together brown sugar, corn syrup, and margarine. Place the pan in the oven for 5 minutes. Stir the mixture until it is well mixed. It will be sticky and thick.
2. Using a sharp paring knife, cut the rind and pith away from the oranges. Slice oranges crosswise into 1/4-inch thick slices. Place the slices in a single layer in the bottom of the pan.
3. In a bowl and using a whisk or electric mixer, beat sugar, orange rind, yogurt, orange juice, oil, egg, and egg whites.
4. In another bowl, stir together flour, baking powder, and salt. With a wooden spoon, stir the dry ingredients into the orange mixture just until everything is combined. Pour the mixture into the pan.
5. Place the pan in the centre of the oven and bake for 30 minutes or until a tester comes out dry.
6. Let the pan cool on a wire rack for 20 minutes. Carefully invert the cake onto a serving platter.

carrot cake with cream cheese frosting

My favourite cake from my first cookbook, *Toronto's Dessert Scene*, was the Carrot Cake given to me by Carole Ogus, from Carole's Cheesecake. It is fabulous but loaded with fat and calories. This version greatly reduces the fat by replacing a lot of the oil or butter with pineapple, more carrots, and low-fat yogurt. The icing uses a small amount of low-fat cream cheese and spreads nicely over the cake.

CAKE

1/3 cup margarine or
    butter

1 cup granulated sugar

2 large eggs

1 tsp vanilla

1 large ripe banana,
    mashed

2 cups grated carrots

2/3 cup raisins

1/2 cup canned crushed
    pineapple, drained

1/2 cup low-fat yogurt

2 cups all-purpose flour

1 1/2 tsp baking powder

1 1/2 tsp baking soda

1 1/2 tsp ground cinnamon

1/4 tsp ground nutmeg

ICING

1/3 cup light cream cheese,
    softened

2/3 cup icing sugar

1 tbsp low-fat milk or water

Preheat the oven to 350°F. Spray a 9-inch Bundt pan with vegetable spray.

1. Make cake: In a large bowl, cream together margarine and sugar until they are smooth; add eggs and vanilla, and beat the mixture well (the mixture may look curdled). Add banana, carrots, raisins, pineapple, and yogurt; stir until everything is well combined.
2. In a bowl, stir together flour, baking powder, baking soda, cinnamon, and nutmeg until combined. Add them to the carrot mixture; stir just until everything is combined. Pour the mixture into a prepared pan.
3. Place the pan in the centre of the oven and bake for 40 to 45 minutes or until a tester inserted in the centre comes out clean. Let the pan cool for 10 minutes before inverting the cake onto a serving plate.
4. Make icing: In a bowl or food processor, beat together cream cheese, icing sugar, and milk until the mixture is smooth; drizzle it over top of the cake. Decorate with grated carrots if desired.

MAKES 16 SERVINGS

NUTRITIONAL ANALYSIS
PER SERVING

Energy 223 calories

Protein 4 g

Fat, total 5 g

Fat, saturated 1 g

Carbohydrates 41 g

Fibre 1 g

Cholesterol 30 mg

NUTRITION WATCH

People often think carrot cake is healthier than other desserts. Not so! Most of these cakes use a batter made of oil, butter, eggs, and regular sour cream, and icing based on butter or vegetable shortening. Be careful of recipes that sound healthy!

TIPS

Very ripe bananas can be kept frozen for up to 1 year.

Raisins can be replaced with chopped, pitted dates, apricots, or prunes.

Use a food processor to mix the batter but take care not to overprocess it.

date cake with coconut topping

MAKES 16 SERVINGS

NUTRITIONAL ANALYSIS
PER SERVING
Energy 217 calories
Protein 3 g
Fat, total 5 g
Fat, saturated 2 g
Carbohydrates 41 g
Fibre 2 g
Cholesterol 27 mg

NUTRITION WATCH
Dates are often used in
desserts to lower the fat.
They have a buttery taste
when puréed and give the
cake the moisture that fat
would supply. They are a
good source of protein and
iron, too.

TIPS
To chop dates easily, use
kitchen shears.

Whole pitted dates can be
used; use a food processor
to mash them after they are
cooked.

Try chopped, pitted prunes
instead of dates.

Cooking dates so they soften to the point where they become a purée makes a great addition to a dessert, because it gives flavour and moisture. This cake is outstanding with the coconut topping, which enhances the cake.

CAKE
12 oz (2 1/2 cups) chopped, pitted
   dried dates
1 3/4 cups water
1/4 cup margarine or butter
1 cup granulated sugar
2 large eggs
1 1/2 cups all-purpose flour
1 1/2 tsp baking powder
1 tsp baking soda

TOPPING
1/3 cup unsweetened coconut
1/4 cup packed brown sugar
3 tbsp low-fat milk
2 tbsp margarine or butter

Preheat the oven to 350°F. Spray a 9-inch square cake pan with vegetable spray.

1. Make cake: Place the dates and water in a saucepan; bring them to a boil, cover, and reduce the heat to low. Cook for 10 minutes, stirring often, or until the dates are soft and most of the liquid has been absorbed. Set the pan aside to cool for 10 minutes.
2. In a large bowl or food processor, beat together the margarine and sugar. Add the eggs and mix well. Add the cooled date mixture and mix everything well.
3. In a bowl, combine flour, baking powder, and baking soda. Stir the dry ingredients into the date mixture just until everything is blended. Pour the mixture into a prepared pan.
4. Place the pan in the centre of the oven and bake for 35 to 40 minutes or until a tester inserted in the centre comes out dry. Let the pan cool on a wire rack.
4. Make topping: In a small saucepan, combine the coconut, brown sugar, milk, and margarine; cook the mixture over medium heat, stirring, for 2 minutes, or until the sugar dissolves. Pour the topping over the cake.

brownie fudge cake

You can tell that I love chocolate desserts. This one has a combination of a brownie and cake and is moist and delicious.

CAKE

1/4 cup semi-sweet chocolate chips

2 tbsp water

1 cup granulated sugar

1/2 cup unsweetened cocoa powder

1 large egg

2 large egg whites

3/4 cup low-fat sour cream

1/2 cup corn syrup

1/4 cup vegetable oil

2 tsp vanilla

1 1/4 cups all-purpose flour

1 1/2 tsp baking powder

ICING

2/3 cup icing sugar

1 tbsp unsweetened cocoa powder

5 tsp water

Preheat the oven to 350°F. Spray a 9-inch square baking pan with vegetable spray.

1. Make cake: In small microwavable bowl, combine the chocolate chips and water. Cook on high for 30 seconds or just until the chips begin to melt. Stir the mixture until it is smooth.
2. In a large bowl and using a whisk or electric mixer, beat sugar, cocoa, egg, egg whites, sour cream, corn syrup, oil, vanilla, and melted chocolate.
3. In another bowl, stir together the flour and baking powder. With a wooden spoon, stir the dry ingredients into the sour cream mixture just until everything is combined. Pour the mixture into a prepared pan.
4. Place the pan in the centre of the oven and bake for 30 to 35 minutes or until a tester comes out dry.
5. Let the pan cool on a wire rack.
6. Make icing: In a bowl and using a whisk or electric mixer, beat icing sugar, cocoa, and water until the mixture is smooth. Spread it over the cake.

MAKES 16 SERVINGS

NUTRITIONAL ANALYSIS PER SERVING

Energy 216 calories

Protein 2.9 g

Fat, total 5.8 g

Fat, saturated 1.6 g

Carbohydrates 38 g

Fibre 1.4 g

Cholesterol 17 mg

NUTRITION WATCH

There is no difference in calories or nutrition between dark or light corn syrup. Dark has a stronger flavour and a darker colour than light corn syrup, which has been clarified to remove all colour and cloudiness.

TIPS

Be sure not to burn your chocolate. If you're uncertain, microwave it on the defrost cycle for a shorter time, just until the chips begin to melt, and check it more often.

If the icing thickens, add a few drops of water or heat it gently in the microwave for 10 seconds.

double chocolate chip banana cake

MAKES 16 SERVINGS

NUTRITIONAL ANALYSIS
PER SERVING

Energy 270 calories

Protein 3.7 g

Fat, total 7.5 g

Fat, saturated 2.2 g

Carbohydrates 63 g

Fibre 2.2 g

Cholesterol 30 mg

NUTRITION WATCH

Zucchini is an extremely
low-fat vegetable. Like the
banana and pineapple in this
recipe, it adds moisture to the
recipe without adding fat.

TIPS

The surprise ingredient here
is zucchini, which gives
incredible moisture to the
cake. Carrots work well, too.

Freeze overripe bananas in
their skins for up to 1 year.
Defrost and use them mashed
in baking.

Try it without the icing— it's
delicious either way.

This has to be the best chocolate cake I've ever baked. The combination of fruit and vegetables keeps it moist, and the cocoa and sprinkling of chocolate chips give it a dense chocolate flavour.

CAKE

1 cup packed brown sugar

1/2 cup granulated sugar

1/3 cup vegetable oil

1 ripe (1/3 cup) medium banana, mashed

1 tsp vanilla

2 large eggs

2 cups finely chopped or grated peeled zucchini

1/2 cup canned crushed pineapple, drained

2 cups all-purpose flour

1/3 cup unsweetened cocoa powder

1 1/2 tsp baking powder

1 1/2 tsp baking soda

1/3 cup semi-sweet chocolate chips

1/4 cup low-fat sour cream

CHOCOLATE CREAM CHEESE ICING

1/3 cup light cream cheese, softened

1 cup icing sugar

1 tbsp unsweetened cocoa powder

1 tbsp low-fat milk

Preheat the oven to 350°F. Spray a 12-cup Bundt pan with vegetable spray.

1. Make cake: In a food processor, combine brown sugar, granulated sugar, oil, banana, vanilla, and eggs; process the mixture until it is smooth. Add zucchini and pineapple; process the mixture just until everything is combined.

2. In a bowl, stir together flour, cocoa, baking powder, and baking soda. Stir the wet ingredients into dry ingredients just until they are mixed. Stir in the chocolate chips and sour cream. Spoon the mixture into a prepared pan.

3. Place the pan in the centre of the oven and bake 40 to 45 minutes or until a tester inserted in the centre comes out clean. Let the pan cool on a wire rack.

4. Make icing: With an electric mixer or food processor, cream together cream cheese, icing sugar, cocoa, and milk. Spread mixture over the cooled cake.

milk chocolate fudge cake

This is a dense chocolate cake that tastes so heavenly, you'll never believe it's low in fat. I love to serve it with a chocolate or raspberry sauce (see Sauces).

1/2 cup milk chocolate chips
3 tbsp water
1 tbsp chocolate liqueur
3/4 cup granulated sugar
1/2 cup unsweetened cocoa powder
3 tbsp all-purpose flour
2 large egg yolks
3/4 cup evaporated skim milk
2 large egg whites
1/4 tsp cream of tartar
3 tbsp granulated sugar

Preheat the oven to 350°F. Spray a 8-inch springform pan with vegetable spray.

1. In a small microwavable bowl, combine chocolate chips, water, and liqueur. Microwave the mixture on high for 40 seconds. Stir it until it is smooth.
2. In a large bowl, whisk together 3/4 cup sugar, cocoa, flour, egg yolks, and evaporated milk. Whisk in the chocolate mixture.
3. In another bowl, beat the egg whites with the cream of tartar until they are foamy. Gradually add 3 tbsp sugar, beating until stiff peaks form. Fold the mixture into the batter just until blended. Pour the batter into a prepared pan.
4. Place the pan in the centre of the oven and bake for 30 to 35 minutes or until the cake is just set at the centre.
5. Let the pan cool on a wire rack. Chill.

MAKES 12 SERVINGS

NUTRITIONAL ANALYSIS
PER SERVING
Energy 150 calories
Protein 3.5 g
Fat, total 3.5 g
Fat, saturated 1.8 g
Carbohydrates 26 g
Fibre 1.7 g
Cholesterol 36 mg

NUTRITION WATCH
All chocolate, whether it's white, dark, or milk chocolate, has approximately the same amount of fat and calories. One ounce has about 130 calories and 9 g of fat.

TIP
Be sure you don't burn chocolate when melting it in the microwave. Always err on the side of caution and microwave for less time if you're uncertain.

molasses and ginger chiffon cake

MAKES 12 SERVINGS

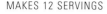

NUTRITIONAL ANALYSIS
PER SERVING

Energy 169 calories

Protein 3.3 g

Fat, total 4.4 g

Fat, saturated 0.5 g

Carbohydrates 29 g

Fibre 0.8 g

Cholesterol 35 mg

NUTRITION WATCH

The traditional chiffon cakes
sound like they are low in fat,
but most have as many as
6 egg yolks, which add greatly
to the fat and cholesterol.
This version only uses two,
with more whites. You won't
notice the difference.

TIP

When beating egg whites,
always make sure that the
beaters and bowls are dry
and clean. Any foreign material can prevent the whites
from foaming completely.
If this does happen, try
adding 1 tsp of lemon juice
to every 3 egg whites and
continue beating.

Chiffon cakes have a lovely light texture, usually from lots of egg yolks and egg whites.
This heavenly one relies upon egg white for its airiness.

1 tbsp instant coffee granules

3 tbsp hot water

3/4 cup granulated sugar

3/4 tsp ground ginger

2 large egg yolks

1/4 cup molasses

3 tbsp vegetable oil

6 (approximately 2/3 cup) large egg whites

1/2 tsp cream of tartar

1/3 cup granulated sugar

1 cup cake and pastry flour

1 1/2 tsp baking powder

Preheat the oven to 325°F. Use a 10-inch tube pan, ungreased.

1. Dissolve the instant coffee in hot water.
2. In a large bowl, whisk together 3/4 cup sugar, ginger, egg yolks, molasses, oil, and cooled coffee.
3. In another bowl, beat the egg whites with the cream of tartar until they are foamy. Gradually add
   1/3 cup sugar, beating until stiff peaks form.
4. Into a separate bowl, sift the flour with the baking powder. Gently fold the dry ingredients into
   the molasses mixture. Gently fold in the egg whites. Pour the mixture into a pan.
5. Place the pan in the centre of the oven and bake for 30 to 35 minutes or until a tester comes out
   dry. Invert the cake immediately onto a wire rack, taking care so that the cake does not crack,
   and let it rest until it is completely cool. Take the cake out of the pan carefully, using a knife to
   separate it from the sides of pan.

gingerbread cake with molasses cream cheese frosting

Gingerbread, whether in a cookie, cake, or any dessert, has a unique combination of flavours. The molasses, cinnamon, and ginger give it that distinctness.

CAKE
1 cup packed brown sugar
1 tsp ground cinnamon
1/2 tsp ground ginger
1 large egg
2 large egg whites
3/4 cup low-fat yogurt
1/2 cup molasses
3 tbsp vegetable oil
1 1/3 cups all-purpose flour
1 tsp baking powder
1/2 tsp baking soda

FROSTING
2 oz light cream cheese, softened
1/3 cup icing sugar
2 tsp molasses
1 1/2 tsp water

Preheat the oven to 350°F. Spray a 13-inch × 9-inchcake pan with vegetable spray.

1. Make cake: In a large bowl and using a whisk or electric mixer, beat brown sugar, cinnamon, ginger, egg, egg whites, yogurt, molasses, and oil.
2. In another bowl, stir together flour, baking powder, and baking soda. With a wooden spoon, stir the dry ingredients into the molasses mixture just until everything is combined. Pour the mixture into a prepared pan.
3. Place the pan in the centre of the oven and bake for 20 to 25 minutes or until a tester comes out dry.
4. Let the pan cool on a wire rack.
5. Make frosting: Using a food processor or electric mixer, beat the cream cheese, icing sugar, molasses, and water until the mixture is smooth. Spread it over the cooled cake.

MAKES 16 SERVINGS

NUTRITIONAL ANALYSIS PER SERVING
Energy 178 calories
Protein 2.9 g
Fat, total 3.8 g
Fat, saturated 0.8 g
Carbohydrates 33 g
Fibre 0.4 g
Cholesterol 16 mg

NUTRITION WATCH
Molasses is rich in iron, calcium, and phosphorous. Be sure to buy dark molasses for your baking. Contrary to belief, blackstrap is only marginally more nutritious than regular molasses.

TIP
If your brown sugar becomes hard, try microwaving it for a few seconds and then add a piece of bread to your container. That always keeps it moist.

maple apple cinnamon cake

MAKES 16 SERVINGS

NUTRITIONAL ANALYSIS
PER SERVING
Energy 218 calories
Protein 2.9 g
Fat, total 5.2 g
Fat, saturated 0.5 g
Carbohydrates 40 g
Fibre 0.8 g
Cholesterol 14 mg

NUTRITION WATCH
Applesauce is simply cooked
and puréed apples. It is a
wonderful low-fat ingredient
to use in baking as a substitute for some of the fat. You
can reduce the fat by as much
as 75% by using applesauce,
or another cooked puréed
fruit.

TIPS
Be sure to buy unsweetened
applesauce, and choose small
jars because the sauce goes
bad quickly after opening.

Always use a clean utensil in
the jar to keep out bacteria.

This cake resembles a light apple coffee cake. The applesauce sweetens the cake as well as giving it moisture, so you don't need much fat.

CAKE
1/2 cup packed brown sugar
1 tsp ground cinnamon
1 large egg
2 large egg whites
1 cup unsweetened applesauce
1/2 cup maple syrup
1/2 cup low-fat yogurt
1/3 cup vegetable oil
2 tsp vanilla
2 cups all-purpose flour

1 1/2 tsp baking powder
1 tsp baking soda
1 cup diced, peeled apples
2 tbsp granulated sugar
1 tbsp all-purpose flour

ICING
1 cup icing sugar
2 tbsp maple syrup
1 tbsp water

Preheat the oven to 350°F. Spray a 9-inch Bundt pan with vegetable spray.

1. Make cake: In a large bowl and using a whisk or electric mixer, beat together brown sugar, cinnamon, egg, egg whites, applesauce, maple syrup, yogurt, oil, and vanilla.
2. In another bowl, stir together 2 cups flour, baking powder, and baking soda. With a wooden spoon, stir the dry ingredients into the applesauce mixture just until everything is combined.
3. In another bowl, toss together apples, sugar, and 1 tbsp flour. Stir the mixture into the batter. Pour it into a prepared pan.
4. Place the pan in the centre of the oven and bake for 35 to 40 minutes or until a tester comes out dry.
5. Let the pan cool on a wire rack.
6. Make icing: In a bowl and using an electric mixer, beat together the icing sugar, syrup, and water. Add additional water as needed to achieve spreading consistency. Spread the icing over the cake.

pumpkin orange maple cake

The combination of orange, pumpkin, and maple syrup is fabulous in this snacking cake.
I pack these squares in the kids' lunches.

CAKE
1 cup packed brown sugar

1 1/2 tsp ground cinnamon

1/4 tsp ground ginger

1 large egg

2 oz light cream cheese, softened

1/2 cup pumpkin purée

1/2 cup low-fat yogurt

2 tsp finely grated orange rind

1/3 cup fresh orange juice

1/4 cup vegetable oil

3 tbsp maple syrup

1 1/2 cups all-purpose flour

1 1/2 tsp baking powder

1/2 tsp baking soda

2 large egg whites

1/4 tsp cream of tartar

1/4 cup granulated sugar

ICING
1/2 cup icing sugar

2 tbsp maple syrup

1 1/2 tsp water

Preheat the oven to 350°F. Spray a 9-inch square cake pan with vegetable spray.

1. Make cake: In a large bowl and using a whisk or electric mixer, beat brown sugar, cinnamon, ginger, egg, cream cheese, pumpkin purée, yogurt, orange rind, orange juice, oil, and maple syrup.
2. In another bowl, stir together the flour, baking powder, and baking soda. With a wooden spoon, stir the dry ingredients into the pumpkin mixture just until everything is combined.
3. In a separate bowl and using clean beaters, beat the egg whites with the cream of tartar until they are foamy. Gradually add the sugar, beating until stiff peaks form. Stir one quarter of the egg whites into the batter. Gently fold in the remaining egg whites just until blended. Pour the mixture into a prepared pan.
4. Place the pan in the centre of the oven and bake for 35 minutes or until a tester comes out dry.
5. Let the pan cool on a wire rack.
6. Make icing: In a bowl and using an electric mixer, beat icing sugar, maple syrup, and water. Spread the mixture over top of the cooled cake.

orange poppyseed bundt cake

MAKES 14 SERVINGS

NUTRITIONAL ANALYSIS
PER SERVING
Energy 213 calories
Protein 4.6 g
Fat, total 6.9 g
Fat, saturated 1.6 g
Carbohydrates 32 g
Fibre 0.3 g
Cholesterol 20 mg

NUTRITION WATCH
Light cream cheese is
reduced by 25% fat from
regular cream cheese, which
has 35% fat. It is not a
low-fat product, so use it
carefully.

TIP
Be sure to beat the ricotta
mixture well to get it as
smooth as possible. A food
processor lets you achieve a
good consistency.

This is a dense orange coffee cake, delicious with a strong citrus flavour.

CAKE
1 1/3 cups granulated sugar
2 large eggs
1 cup smooth 5% ricotta cheese
2/3 cup low-fat yogurt
1/3 cup vegetable oil
3 tbsp orange juice concentrate
1 tbsp finely grated orange rind
1 1/3 cups all-purpose flour
2 1/4 tsp baking powder
2 tsp poppyseeds
1/2 tsp baking soda

ICING
2 oz light cream cheese,
  softened
2/3 cup icing sugar
1 tbsp orange juice concentrate

Preheat the oven to 350°F. Spray a 9-inch Bundt pan with vegetable spray.

1. Make cake: In a food processor, combine sugar, eggs, ricotta cheese, yogurt, oil, orange juice concentrate, and orange rind; purée the mixture until it is smooth. Transfer it to a large bowl.
2. In another bowl, stir together flour, baking powder, poppyseeds, and baking soda. With a wooden spoon, stir the dry ingredients into the orange mixture just until everything is combined. Pour the mixture into a prepared pan.
3. Place the pan in the centre of the oven and bake for 30 to 35 minutes or until a tester inserted in the centre comes out clean. Let the pan cool on a wire rack until room temperature.
4. Make icing: Using either a food processor or electric mixer, beat cream cheese, icing sugar, and orange juice concentrate until the mixture is smooth. Drizzle it over the cake.

cobblers, crisps, and crumbles

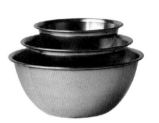

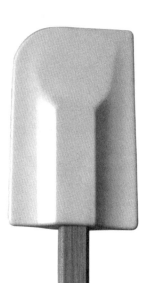

tips for divine light cobblers, crisps, and crumbles

1. A cobbler is a baked deep-dish fruit dessert topped with a thick biscuit crust, often sprinkled with sugar. The toppings in these recipes require little fat because they use yogurt or buttermilk.

2. A cobbler is done when a toothpick or cake tester inserted into the crust comes out dry and clean. It's best served warm with frozen yogurt, fruit sauce, or a vanilla-based sauce (see Sauces). Cobblers are great reheated — just place them in a 350°F oven for 10 minutes.

3. Crisps and crumbles are fruit-based desserts topped with a crumbly mixture often made with rolled oats, low-fat granola, or Grape-Nuts, which is a low-fat wheat and toasted barley cereal.

4. Crisps are done when the topping is browned and crisp and the fruit is tender. They are tasty served warm or at room temperature with either frozen yogurt or Vanilla Cream (see page 241).

5. Either fresh or frozen fruit can be used in cobblers, crisps, or crumbles. Fresh fruit will always taste best, but if you are using frozen, measure it when it is frozen, then defrost it and drain it well before using.

buttermilk cranberry apple cobbler

I love cobblers all year round — even if you don't have fresh fruit, you can always use frozen. Just be sure to thaw and drain it well. My favourite apples are Mutsu, Granny Smith, and Spy because of their taste and texture. Serve this cobbler still hot from the oven, with frozen yogurt.

FILLING

6 cups sliced, peeled apples

1 1/2 cups cranberries

1 cup granulated sugar

3/4 tsp ground cinnamon

1/3 cup apple juice

1 1/2 tbsp cornstarch

TOPPING

3/4 cup all-purpose flour

1/3 cup granulated sugar

1/2 tsp baking powder

1/4 cup buttermilk

1 tbsp vegetable oil

1 large egg

1 tbsp granulated sugar

1/2 tsp ground cinnamon

Preheat oven to 375°F. Spray a 9-inch square cake pan with vegetable spray.

1. Make filling: In a large bowl, stir together apples, cranberries, sugar, and cinnamon. In a small bowl, whisk the apple juice with the cornstarch until smooth; stir the liquid into the fruit mixture. Pour the mixture into a prepared pan.
2. Make topping: In a bowl, stir together flour, 1/3 cup sugar, and baking powder. In another bowl, mix the buttermilk, oil, and egg. With a wooden spoon, add the dry ingredients to the wet and mix until everything is combined. Drop the batter by spoonfuls on top of the fruit mixture.
3. Stir together 1 tbsp sugar and cinnamon; sprinkle the mixture over the batter.
4. Place the pan in the centre of the oven and bake for 40 minutes or until a tester placed in the centre comes out dry. Serve warm.

MAKES 12 SERVINGS

NUTRITIONAL ANALYSIS
PER SERVING

Energy 188 calories

Protein 1.6 g

Fat, total 1.9 g

Fat, saturated 0.3 g

Carbohydrates 41 g

Fibre 1.9 g

Cholesterol 18 mg

NUTRITION WATCH

Apples provide a good source of dietary fibre and carbohydrates. Cranberries are very high in vitamin C. A cobbler is an easy way to get kids to eat more fruit.

TIPS

Feel free to replace the apples with pears for a change.

If you're using frozen cranberries, you don't have to thaw them first.

If you don't have apple juice, try orange juice.

Instead of buttermilk, you can use low-fat yogurt or add 1 tsp lemon juice to 1/4 cup of milk and let stand 5 minutes.

sour cream blueberry peach cobbler

MAKES 12 SERVINGS

NUTRITIONAL ANALYSIS
PER SERVING
Energy 154 calories
Protein 2.3 g
Fat, total 3 g
Fat, saturated 0.8 g
Carbohydrates 2.9 g
Fibre 1.4 g
Cholesterol 20 mg

NUTRITION WATCH
Peaches contain both
vitamins A and C, and potassium. Blueberries are high in
vitamin C and are a good
source of fibre, potassium,
and carbohydrates. Together
they pack a dynamic nutritional punch.

TIPS
If you're using frozen fruit,
measure it when it is still
frozen, then be sure to thaw
and drain well or your cobbler
will be too wet.

If you're using fresh peaches,
make sure you choose ripe
ones.

Blueberries and peaches make a perfect combination in this warm and delicious cobbler. I like to serve this cobbler hot with a scoop of vanilla frozen yogurt or with Vanilla Cream (see page 241).

FILLING	TOPPING
2 1/2 cups blueberries	1 cup all-purpose flour
2 1/2 cups sliced and peeled peaches	1 tsp baking powder
	1/3 cup granulated sugar
1 tbsp cornstarch	1 large egg
1/3 cup granulated sugar	1/3 cup low-fat sour cream
1/4 tsp ground cinnamon	2 tbsp margarine or butter, softened
	1 tbsp water

Preheat oven to 350°F. Spray a 8-inch square cake pan with vegetable spray.

1. Make filling: In a bowl, stir together the blueberries, peaches, and cornstarch.
2. In another bowl, stir together the sugar and cinnamon. Set aside 1 tbsp. Stir the remaining cinnamon sugar into the berry mixture. Pour the mixture into a prepared pan.
3. Make topping: In a bowl, stir together the flour and baking powder. In another bowl, mix the sugar, egg, sour cream, margarine, and water. With a wooden spoon, add the dry ingredients to the wet until everything is combined. Drop by spoonfuls on top of the fruit mixture.
4. Sprinkle with the reserved cinnamon sugar.
5. Place the pan in the centre of the oven and bake for 35 to 40 minutes or until a tester inserted in the centre comes out dry.
6. Serve warm.

rhubarb strawberry granola crisp

Crisps are especially delicious when fruit is fresh and ripe. Serve this crisp with Vanilla Cream (see page 241). The combination of sweet strawberries, tart rhubarb, and a crunchy sweet topping make a unique crisp.

FILLING

2 1/2 cups sliced strawberries

2 cups sliced rhubarb

3/4 cup granulated sugar

1 tbsp cornstarch

TOPPING

3/4 cup all-purpose flour

2/3 cup low-fat granola

1/3 cup packed brown sugar

1/2 tsp ground cinnamon

2 1/2 tbsp water

2 tbsp vegetable oil

Preheat oven to 350°F. Spray a 9-inch square cake pan with vegetable spray.

1. Make filling: In a bowl, stir together strawberries, rhubarb, sugar, and cornstarch. Pour the mixture into a prepared baking dish.
2. Make topping: In another bowl, stir together flour, granola, brown sugar, cinnamon, water, and oil until crumbly. Sprinkle it over the fruit mixture.
3. Place the pan in the centre of the oven for 30 minutes or until the topping is browned and crisp.
4. Serve warm.

MAKES 12 SERVINGS

NUTRITIONAL ANALYSIS
PER SERVING

Energy 165 calories

Protein 1.7 g

Fat, total 2.9 g

Fat, saturated 0.2 g

Carbohydrates 33 g

Fibre 1.8 g

Cholesterol 0 mg

NUTRITION WATCH

Strawberries are an excellent source of vitamin C and also provide potassium, iron, and fibre.

TIPS

Frozen cut-up rhubarb is sold in the supermarket. Measure it when it is still frozen; then thaw it and drain it well.

There are many different varieties of granola in the stores; choose your favourite, but be sure it is low fat.

pear and plum crumble

MAKES 12 SERVINGS

NUTRITIONAL ANALYSIS
PER SERVING

Energy 168 calories

Protein 1.5 g

Fat, total 2.8 g

Fat, saturated 0.2 g

Carbohydrates 34 g

Fibre 1.7 g

Cholesterol 0 mg

NUTRITION WATCH

Pears are a high source of
fibre and potassium. Plums
contain a fair amount of
vitamin A and potassium.

TIPS

Be sure the pears are ripe
and sweet. My favourite
pears are Bartlett and Bosc.

The best plums are Italian
prune plums, which are small
and purple.

Grape-Nuts cereal makes a wonderfully crunchy topping for a crumble. It is a good substitute for chopped nuts, without excess fat and calories. Ripe pears and plums make this crumble a wonderful summer dessert, especially teamed with fruit sorbet.

FILLING	TOPPING
2 cups sliced, peeled pears	2/3 cup packed brown sugar
2 cups sliced plums	1/2 cup all-purpose flour
1/3 cup granulated sugar	1/3 cup Grape-Nuts cereal
1/4 tsp ground cinnamon	1/3 cup quick-cooking oats
1/4 cup orange juice	1/4 tsp ground cinnamon
1 tbsp cornstarch	2 1/2 tbsp water
	2 tbsp vegetable oil

Preheat oven to 350°F. Spray a 8-inch square cake pan with vegetable spray.

1. Make filling: In a bowl, stir together pears, plums, sugar, and cinnamon. In a small bowl, whisk the orange juice with the cornstarch until it is smooth; stir into the fruit mixture. Pour the mixture into a prepared pan.
2. Make topping: In the bowl, stir together brown sugar, flour, cereal, oats, cinnamon, water, and oil until crumbly. Sprinkle it over the fruit mixture.
3. Place the pan in the centre of the oven and bake for 30 to 35 minutes or until the crumble is golden.
4. Serve warm.

strawberry blueberry double crisp

The combination of low-fat granola and the cooking oats makes a light and crispy topping, with a nutty texture without excess fat and calories.

1 1/2 cups blueberries
1 1/2 cups sliced strawberries
1/4 cup granulated sugar
1 tbsp all-purpose flour
1 cup all-purpose flour
3/4 cup packed brown sugar
3/4 cup quick-cooking oats
1/2 cup low-fat granola
1 tsp ground cinnamon
1/4 cup vegetable oil
2 tbsp water

Preheat oven to 350°F. Spray a 8-inch square cake pan with vegetable spray.

1. In bowl, stir together blueberries, strawberries, sugar, and 1 tbsp flour.
2. In another bowl, stir together 1 cup flour, brown sugar, oats, granola, and cinnamon. Stir in the oil and water until the mixture is crumbly. Pat half of it into a prepared baking dish. Pour the berry mixture evenly over top. Sprinkle the remaining oat mixture on top.
3. Place the pan in the centre of the oven and bake for 25 minutes or until the crisp is golden.

MAKES 12 SERVINGS

NUTRITIONAL ANALYSIS
PER SERVING
Energy 207 calories
Protein 2.6 g
Fat, total 5.4 g
Fat, saturated 0.4 g
Carbohydrates 37 g
Fibre 1.9 g
Cholesterol 0 mg

NUTRITION WATCH
Granola cereals may sound healthy, but most are loaded with fat, sugar, and lots of calories. Low-fat versions are delicious and use much less fat and sugar.

TIP
If you're using frozen berries, measure them when they're still frozen, and then thaw and drain them well.

pies, flans, and tarts

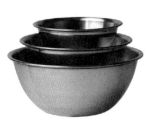

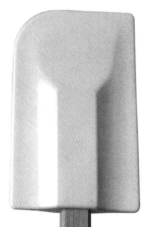

tips for divine light pies, flans, and tarts

1. All the pie recipes in this chapter use a standard 9-inch pie plate, either glass or metal. I always spray the plate with vegetable spray. Flan dishes are metal and come in 8-inch or 9-inch sizes; they have fluted edges and a removable bottom, which makes a very attractive dessert.

2. The best low-fat crusts are made with cookie crumbs (either graham, chocolate wafers, or vanilla crumbs) or are a baked crust made with an egg-white meringue. Crumb crusts are held together with a small amount of oil or butter and water or honey, and are always patted on the bottom and side of the pan.

3. Some recipes have pie crust made from butter, oil, light cream cheese, and yogurt or water. This crust must be rolled into a ball and chilled for 20 minutes, then rolled out between waxed paper and fitted into the pie plate. This delicious crust contains very little fat compared to a regular pie crust.

4. Gelatin is used in several of the mousse pie recipes. One package of unflavoured gelatin powder equals approximately 1 tbsp. Add 2 to 3 tbsp of cold water and let it sit for 2 minutes. Then either add 1 tbsp of hot water or microwave the mixture just until the gelatin dissolves, approximately 20 seconds. Stir until it is well mixed.

5. When you're beating egg whites, always be sure that the bowl and beaters are dry and clean, or the egg whites will not beat to their proper volume. If the egg whites do not beat properly, add 2 tsp lemon juice for every 3 egg whites. Fold the whites gently into the batter just until they are incorporated.

6. A baked pie is ready when the centre is still slightly loose. Let it cool to room temperature and then chill before serving.

7. Pie fillings can include such ingredients as low-fat ricotta cheese, which takes the place of regular cream cheese, or low-fat yogurt or sour cream, which can take the place of regular sour cream. Evaporated skim milk and low-fat condensed milk replace heavy cream.

8. Garnish pies, flans, and tarts with icing sugar or cocoa. Make spider or spiral designs on top using melted chocolate or a combination of low-fat sour cream mixed with a little water and sugar. Put the mixture in a small plastic bag, then cut the very tip of the end off. Draw four concentric circles on top of the pie filling before baking and run a toothpick through the circles at regular intervals.

pecan cream cheese pie

The combination of cheesecake and pecan is too good for words. I like to serve this pie either at room temperature or chilled.

CRUST
1 1/2 cups vanilla wafer crumbs
2 tbsp granulated sugar
2 tbsp water
1 tbsp vegetable oil

CHEESECAKE FILLING
3/4 cup smooth 5% ricotta cheese
1/3 cup granulated sugar
1/3 cup light cream cheese
1/4 cup light sour cream
1 large egg
1 tbsp all-purpose flour
1 tsp vanilla

PECAN FILLING
2/3 cup packed brown sugar
1/2 cup chopped pecans
1 large egg
2 large egg whites
1/2 cup corn syrup
1 tbsp molasses

Preheat the oven to 375°F. Spray a 9-inch pie plate with vegetable spray.

1. Make crust: Mix the crumbs, sugar, water, and oil together until the mixture holds together. Press it into the side and bottom of a pie plate. Bake for 8 minutes.
2. Make cheesecake filling: In a food processor, purée the ricotta cheese, sugar, cream cheese, sour cream, egg, flour, and vanilla until the mixture is smooth. Pour it into the pie crust.
3. Make pecan filling: In a bowl, whisk together the brown sugar, pecans, egg, egg whites, corn syrup, and molasses. Pour the mixture carefully over the cheesecake layer.
4. Place the plate in the centre of the oven and bake for approximately 30 to 35 minutes or until the filling is almost set. It may rise up around the edges or even through the middle of the pecan filling.
5. Let the plate cool on a wire rack.

MAKES 12 SERVINGS

NUTRITIONAL ANALYSIS
PER SERVING
Energy 290 calories
Protein 5.1 g
Fat, total 10 g
Fat, saturated 2.9 g
Carbohydrates 46 g
Fibre 0.7 g
Cholesterol 48 mg

NUTRITION WATCH
Pecans are a good source of protein and a healthy polyunsaturated fat. But nuts are high in calories and fat grams, so eat them in moderation, or as an alternative source of protein in your diet.

TIPS
Be sure to process the cheesecake batter well to make as it as smooth as possible.

Pay attention when pouring the pecan layer on top of the cheesecake so they don't mix.

banana cream pie

Banana mousse with a chocolate crust and layered sautéed bananas are the best combination possible. You'd never believe that this pie was lower-fat.

MAKES 12 SERVINGS

NUTRITIONAL ANALYSIS
PER SERVING

Energy 239 calories

Protein 5.2 g

Fat, total 6.9 g

Fat, saturated 2.1 g

Carbohydrates 39 g

Fibre 1.1 g

Cholesterol 7.7 mg

NUTRITION WATCH

Bananas are high in carbohydrates, and rich in
potassium and vitamin C.

TIP

Use ripe bananas for the
best flavour. To ripen
bananas, place them in a
perforated paper bag for a
couple of days.

CRUST

1 3/4 cups chocolate wafer crumbs

2 tbsp granulated sugar

2 1/2 tbsp water

1 tbsp vegetable oil

FILLING

2 tsp margarine or butter

1/4 cup packed brown sugar

2 ripe (3/4 cup) medium
   bananas, sliced

2/3 cup smooth 5% ricotta cheese

2 oz light cream cheese, softened

1/2 cup granulated sugar

2/3 cup low-fat yogurt

1 1/2 tsp vanilla

1/8 tsp salt

2 tsp unflavoured gelatin powder

3 tbsp cold water

2 large egg whites

1/4 tsp cream of tartar

1/4 cup granulated sugar

Spray a 9-inch pie plate with vegetable spray.

1. Make crust: In a bowl, stir together wafer crumbs, sugar, water, and oil. Set aside 1 tbsp of the mixture. Pat the remaining mixture onto the bottom and up the side of a prepared pan.

2. Make filling: In a frying pan, melt the margarine over medium heat. Stir in the brown sugar and bananas; cook for 2 minutes. Pour the mixture evenly into the crust.

3. In a food processor, combine ricotta cheese, cream cheese, 1/2 cup sugar, yogurt, vanilla, and salt; purée the mixture until it is smooth. In a small microwavable bowl, combine the gelatin and water and let it sit for 2 minutes; microwave on high for 20 seconds. Stir the mixture until it is dissolved. With the food processor running, add the gelatin through the feed tube. Transfer the mixture to a large bowl.

4. In another bowl, beat the egg whites with the cream of tartar until they are foamy. Gradually add 1/4 cup sugar, beating until stiff peaks form. Stir one quarter of the egg whites into the ricotta mixture. Gently fold in the remaining egg whites just until blended. Pour the mixture into the crust. Sprinkle with the reserved crumb mixture. Chill for 2 hours or until set.

coconut cream pie

Coconut cream pie is usually avoided by people looking for lighter desserts because coconut milk is a highly saturated fat. Not here! The newest addition to the grocery store is light coconut milk, which is 75% reduced in fat and calories.

CRUST
1 1/2 cups graham crumbs
1/4 cup granulated sugar
1 tbsp toasted coconut
3 tbsp water
1 tbsp vegetable oil

FILLING
1/2 cup granulated sugar
1/2 cup smooth 5% ricotta cheese

2/3 cup light coconut milk
2 oz light cream cheese, softened
2 tsp vanilla
2 tsp unflavoured gelatin powder
2 tbsp cold water
1/4 cup toasted coconut
2 large egg whites
1/4 tsp cream of tartar
1/4 cup granulated sugar

Preheat the oven to 400°F. Spray a 9-inch pie plate with vegetable spray.

1. Make crust: In a bowl, stir together crumbs, sugar, coconut, water, and oil until mixed. Pat the mixture onto the bottom and up the side of a prepared pan. Place the pan in the centre of the oven and bake for 10 minutes or until the crust is slightly browned. Let the pan cool on a wire rack.

2. Make filling: In a food processor, combine 1/2 cup sugar, ricotta cheese, coconut milk, cream cheese, and vanilla; purée the mixture until it is smooth. In a small microwavable bowl, combine the gelatin and water and let it sit for 2 minutes; microwave the mixture on high for 20 seconds. Stir until it is dissolved. With the food processor running, add the gelatin through the feed tube. Transfer the mixture to a large bowl and stir in 3 tbsp toasted coconut.

3. In another bowl, beat the egg whites with the cream of tartar until they are foamy. Gradually add 1/4 cup sugar, beating until stiff peaks form. Gently fold the mixture into the ricotta mixture just until combined and pour it into the crust. Sprinkle remaining toasted coconut over top. Chill for 2 hours or until the filling is set firm.

MAKES 12 SERVINGS

NUTRITIONAL ANALYSIS
PER SERVING
Energy 193 calories
Protein 4.2 g
Fat, total 6.2 g
Fat, saturated 3 g
Carbohydrates 30 g
Fibre 0.9 g
Cholesterol 6.1 mg

NUTRITION WATCH
Coconut is high in potassium, but also high in saturated fat. I only use it in a small amounts and stick to light coconut milk.

TIP
To toast coconut, put it in a skillet over medium heat and toast until it is lightly browned, approximately 2 minutes. Be careful not to burn it!

key lime pie

NUTRITIONAL ANALYSIS
PER SERVING
Energy 277 calories
Protein 6.8 g
Fat, total 6.9 g
Fat, saturated 3 g
Carbohydrates 47 g
Fibre 0.5 g
Cholesterol 16 mg

NUTRITION WATCH
Key lime pie is often made
with butter and whipping
cream. This version uses low-
fat condensed milk, which is
available at most grocery
stores, and the combination
of ricotta and light cream
cheese heavily reduces the
fat and calories.

TIP
To get the most juice from
limes, first be sure that they
are ripe. Roll them firmly on
the kitchen counter, which
helps to release the juices,
or microwave them for
approximately 20 seconds.

Key lime refers to a type of lime that comes from Florida. The type that is most commonly available is actually the Persian lime. But you might not recognize the dessert if I called it Persian Lime Pie! With either type of lime, this is a creamy tart pie.

CRUST
1 1/2 cups graham crumbs
3 tbsp granulated sugar
2 tbsp water
1 tbsp vegetable oil

FILLING
1 can (14 oz) low-fat sweetened
    condensed milk
1/2 cup smooth 5% ricotta
    cheese
4 oz light cream cheese, softened
1/3 cup fresh lime juice
    (approximately 2 limes)
2 tsp finely grated lime rind
1/4 cup granulated sugar

Preheat the oven to 375°F. Spray a 9-inch pie plate with vegetable spray.

1. Make crust: In a bowl, stir together the graham crumbs, sugar, water, and oil until mixed. Pat the mixture onto the bottom and up the side of a prepared pan.
2. Make filling: In a food processor, combine the condensed milk, ricotta cheese, cream cheese, lemon juice and rind, and sugar; purée the mixture until it is smooth. Pour it into the crust.
3. Place the pan in the centre of the oven and bake for approximately 20 minutes or just until the filling is set. Let the pan cool on a wire rack.
4. Chill before serving.

chocolate mud pie

This mud pie tastes so rich you'll think it has a pound of chocolate in it. I like to serve this with a raspberry or chocolate sauce (see Sauces).

CRUST

1 1/2 cups chocolate wafer crumbs

2 tbsp packed brown sugar

2 tbsp water

1 tbsp vegetable oil

FILLING

2 tbsp semi-sweet chocolate chips

1 tbsp water

1 tsp instant coffee granules

1 tbsp hot water

1 1/4 cups packed brown sugar

1/2 cup unsweetened cocoa powder

1 tbsp all-purpose flour

2 1/2 oz light cream cheese, softened

1 large egg

2 large egg whites

1/4 cup low-fat sour cream

3 tbsp corn syrup

1 tsp vanilla

Preheat the oven to 350°F. Spray a 9-inch pie plate with vegetable spray.

1. Make crust: In a bowl, stir together the wafer crumbs, brown sugar, water, and oil until mixed. Pat the mixture onto the bottom and up the side of a prepared pan.
2. Make filling: In a small microwavable bowl, combine the chocolate chips and water. Microwave on high for approximately 30 seconds, or just until the chips begin to melt. Stir the mixture until it is smooth. Cool.
3. Dissolve the instant coffee granules in hot water. Cool.
4. In a food processor, combine the brown sugar, cocoa, flour, cream cheese, egg, egg whites, sour cream, corn syrup, vanilla, chocolate, and coffee; purée the mixture until it is smooth. Pour it into the crust.
5. Place the pan in the centre of the oven and bake for 25 to 30 minutes or until the centre is just set. Let the pan cool on a wire rack. Chill for 1 hour.

MAKES 12 SERVINGS

NUTRITIONAL ANALYSIS PER SERVING

Energy 244 calories

Protein 3.8 g

Fat, total 6.2 g

Fat, saturated 2.1 g

Carbohydrates 45 g

Fibre 1.8 g

Cholesterol 23 mg

NUTRITION WATCH

Chocolate and cocoa differ greatly in fat and calories. Each ounce of chocolate contains 14 g of fat and 140 calories. For each ounce of cocoa, there are 40 calories and 1 g of fat!

TIP

Be careful not to burn the chocolate in the microwave. It's safest to use the defrost cycle, although it takes longer. Always use less time to be certain.

orange chocolate marble pie

Orange and chocolate are wonderful flavours together. The swirled marble top makes this pie look as good as it tastes.

MAKES 12 SERVINGS

NUTRITIONAL ANALYSIS
PER SERVING

Energy 204 calories

Protein 3.7 g

Fat, total 5.5 g

Fat, saturated 1.5 g

Carbohydrates 35 g

Fibre 0.8 g

Cholesterol 21 mg

NUTRITION WATCH

The small amount of chocolate used here does not add
much to the calorie and fat
count of each serving. One
tablespoon of chocolate chips
has approximately 80 calories
and 8 g of fat.

TIP

Be sure to use orange
juice concentrate — not just
orange juice — for the most
intense flavour. Keep a can
in the freezer just for baking
and cooking purposes.

CRUST

1 3/4 cups chocolate
  wafer crumbs

2 tbsp granulated sugar

2 1/2 tbsp water

1 tbsp vegetable oil

FILLING

3/4 cup granulated sugar

2 tbsp all-purpose flour

1/2 cup evaporated
  skim milk

1/2 cup low-fat sour cream

1/4 cup orange juice
  concentrate

2 tsp finely grated orange rind

1 large egg

2 large egg whites

MARBLE

1 tbsp semi-sweet chocolate
  chips

1 1/2 tsp water

Preheat the oven to 375°F. Spray a 9-inch pie plate with vegetable spray.

1. Make crust: In a bowl, stir together the wafer crumbs, sugar, water, and oil until combined. Pat the mixture onto the bottom and up the side of a prepared pan.

2. Make filling: In a bowl, whisk together sugar, flour, evaporated milk, sour cream, orange juice concentrate, orange rind, egg, and egg whites until the mixture is smooth. Pour it into the crust.

3. Make marble: In a small microwavable bowl, combine the chocolate chips and water. On high, microwave for approximately 30 seconds or until the chocolate begins to melt. Stir the mixture until it is smooth. Spoon it on top of the filling; using a butter knife, marble the chocolate through the batter.

4. Place the pan in the centre of the oven and bake for 25 to 30 minutes or until the centre is set. Let the pan cool on a wire rack.

orange mousse in meringue shell

A pastry shell made with egg white is very dramatic. Any mousse fillings could fill this meringue. The longer the meringue stays in the oven, the crisper it becomes.

MERINGUE

3 large egg whites

1/4 tsp cream of tartar

3/4 cup granulated sugar

MOUSSE

1 cup smooth 5% ricotta cheese

2 oz light cream cheese, softened

1/2 cup granulated sugar

1/4 cup orange juice concentrate

4 tsp finely grated orange rind

2 tsp unflavoured gelatin powder

2 tbsp cold water

1/2 cup low-fat yogurt

2 large egg whites

Pinch cream of tartar

1/3 cup granulated sugar

Grated orange rind

Preheat the oven to 275°F. Spray a 9-inch glass pie plate with vegetable spray.

1. In a bowl, beat the egg whites with the cream of tartar until they are foamy. Gradually beat in the sugar, beating until stiff peaks form. Spoon the mixture evenly into a pie shell across the bottom and up the sides.
2. Bake in the centre of the oven for 1 hour. Let the pan cool on a wire rack while you prepare the mousse.
3. Make mousse: In a food processor, combine ricotta cheese, cream cheese, 1/2 cup sugar, orange juice concentrate, and orange rind; purée the mixture until it is smooth. In a small microwavable bowl, combine the gelatin and water; let sit for 2 minutes. Microwave on high for 20 seconds. Stir the mixture until it is smooth. With the motor running, add the gelatin and yogurt though the feed tube. Transfer the mixture to a large bowl.
4. In another bowl, beat the egg whites with the cream of tartar until they are foamy. Gradually add 1/3 cup sugar, beating until stiff peaks form. Stir one quarter of the egg whites into the ricotta-gelatin mixture. Gently fold in the remaining egg whites just until combined. Pour the mixture into the pie shell and chill for at least 1 hour.
5. Garnish with orange rind.

lemon sour cream meringue pie

MAKES 12 SERVINGS

NUTRITIONAL ANALYSIS
PER SERVING
Energy 243 calories
Protein 4 g
Fat, total 5.1 g
Fat, saturated 1.6 g
Carbohydrates 43 g
Fibre 0.4 g
Cholesterol 41 mg

NUTRITION WATCH
Lemon meringue pie is
traditionally loaded with
calories, not so much
from the filling, even though
it usually contains butter,
but from the buttery pie crust.
Traditional pie crusts are
loaded with fat.

TIP
When cooking the lemon
filling, after you've added the
eggs keep the temperature
low or the filling will cook
and curdle. Keep whisking!

This version of lemon meringue pie is so unique because the filling is made creamy by the addition of low-fat sour cream, not butter.

PASTRY	FILLING	MERINGUE TOPPING
1/3 cup granulated sugar	1 cup granulated sugar	3 large egg whites
3 tbsp vegetable oil	3 1/2 tbsp cornstarch	1/4 tsp cream of tartar
3 tbsp low-fat yogurt	1 cup low-fat milk	1/3 cup granulated sugar
1 1/2 oz light cream cheese	2 large egg yolks	
1 1/4 cup all-purpose flour	2 tsp finely grated lemon rind	
	1/4 cup fresh lemon juice	
	1/3 cup low-fat sour cream	

Preheat the oven to 425°F. Spray a 9-inch pie plate with vegetable spray.

1. Make pastry: In a food processor, purée the sugar, oil, yogurt, and cream cheese until the mixture is smooth. Add the flour and process on and off until the mixture is crumbly. Roll it into a smooth ball and wrap in plastic wrap. Chill for 20 minutes.
2. Roll the pastry into a circle large enough to fit the plate. Fit it into the plate, working it up the sides. Place a piece of foil over top. Bake in the centre of the oven for 15 minutes. Remove the foil and bake for another 8 to 10 minutes or until it is golden. Let the pan cool on a wire rack.
3. Make filling: Preheat the oven to 400°F. In a saucepan off the heat, whisk together the sugar, cornstarch, and milk, until the mixture is smooth. Bring it to a boil, whisking constantly, until it thickens, approximately 2 to 3 minutes. Remove the pan from the heat. In a bowl, beat the egg yolks; pour half the hot milk mixture into the eggs and mix well. Return the mixture to the saucepan and cook over low heat for 1 minute, stirring, or until the mixture is thickened and bubbling. Remove it from the heat and stir in the lemon rind and lemon juice. Pour the mixture into a bowl and cool for 10 minutes. Whisk in the sour cream. Pour the mixture into the crust.
4. Make meringue topping: In a clean bowl, beat the egg whites with the cream of tartar until they are foamy. Gradually add the sugar, beating until stiff peaks form. Spoon the mixture over the warm filling, spreading it all the way to the pastry. Place the plate in the centre of the oven and bake for 5 to 7 minutes or until it is golden. Let the plate cool on a wire rack.

lemon mousse pie

A creamy lemon filling over a chocolate cookie crust is to-die-for. This pie is sensational.

CRUST
1 3/4 cups chocolate wafer
   crumbs
1 tbsp sugar
1 tbsp vegetable oil
2 tbsp water

MOUSSE
3/4 cup granulated sugar
1/2 cup smooth 5% ricotta
   cheese
2 oz light cream cheese, softened
1 tbsp finely grated lemon rind
1/3 cup fresh lemon juice
2 tsp unflavoured gelatin
   powder
3 tbsp cold water
3 large egg whites
1/4 tsp cream of tartar
1/2 cup granulated sugar

Spray a 9-inch pie plate with vegetable spray.

1. Make crust: In a bowl, mix the crumbs, sugar, oil, and water just until the crumbs come together. Pat the mixture onto the sides and bottom of a pie plate.

2. Make mousse: In a food processor, combine 3/4 cup sugar, ricotta cheese, cream cheese, lemon rind, and lemon juice; purée until the mixture is smooth. In a small microwavable bowl, combine the gelatin and water and let it sit for 2 minutes; microwave on high for 20 seconds. Stir the mixture until it is dissolved. With the food processor running, add the gelatin mixture through the feed tube. Transfer the mixture to a large bowl.

3. In another bowl, beat the egg whites with the cream of tartar until they are foamy. Gradually add 1/2 cup sugar, beating until stiff peaks form. Stir one quarter of the egg whites into the ricotta mixture. Gently fold in the remaining egg whites just until blended. Spoon the mixture into the crust. Chill for 2 hours or until the filling is set firm. Serve garnished with additional lemon rind, if desired.

MAKES 12 SERVINGS

NUTRITIONAL ANALYSIS
PER SERVING
Energy 200 calories
Protein 4.2 g
Fat, total 5.7 g
Fat, saturated 1.7 g
Carbohydrates 33 g
Fibre 0.7 g
Cholesterol 5.8 mg

NUTRITION WATCH
Whipping cream is traditionally used in mousses — and
contains 35% MF. One tablespoon has 50 calories and
5 g of fat. In a traditional
mousse, you'd use 1 to 2 cups
of cream. That's a lot of
calories!

TIP
Ricotta cheese, cream
cheese, and egg whites make
this mousse so light. Be sure
to process the filling well.

peanut butter mousse pie

MAKES 12 SERVINGS

NUTRITIONAL ANALYSIS
PER SERVING
Energy 174 calories
Protein 5.9 g
Fat, total 6.9 g
Fat, saturated 2 g
Carbohydrates 22 g
Fibre 0.5 g
Cholesterol 8.0 mg

NUTRITION WATCH
Peanuts are a monounsatu-
rated fat, which has proven
to be a healthy fat in terms
of lowering blood cholesterol.
But they should be eaten in
moderation because they
have a high number of calories
and grams of fat.

TIP
When buying peanut butter,
choose a pure, smooth one.
The commercial brands are
often filled with icing sugar
and are hydrogenated, making
make them a source of saturated fat.

I never thought I could have a peanut butter mousse with a chocolate wafer crust and still call it low fat. You must try this dessert — it's sensational!

CRUST
1 3/4 cups chocolate wafer
   crumbs
2 tbsp granulated sugar
2 tbsp water
1 tbsp vegetable oil

MOUSSE
3/4 cup smooth 5% ricotta
   cheese
2 oz light cream cheese, softened
2/3 cup granulated sugar
1/3 cup smooth peanut butter
1/2 cup low-fat yogurt
2 tsp unflavoured gelatin
   powder
3 tbsp cold water
3 large egg whites
1/4 tsp cream of tartar
1/3 cup granulated sugar

Spray a 9-inch pie plate with vegetable spray.

1. Make crust: In a bowl, stir together the wafer crumbs, sugar, water, and oil until combined. Set aside 1 tbsp of the crumb mixture and pat the remainder onto the bottom and up the side of a prepared pan.
2. Make filling: In a food processor, combine ricotta cheese, cream cheese, 2/3 cup sugar, peanut butter, and yogurt; purée the mixture until it is smooth. In a small microwavable bowl, combine the gelatin and water and let it sit for 2 minutes; microwave on high for 20 seconds. Stir the mixture until it is dissolved. With the food processor running, add the gelatin through the feed tube. Transfer the mixture to a large bowl.
3. In another bowl, beat the egg whites with the cream of tartar until they are foamy. Gradually add 1/3 cup sugar, beating until stiff peaks form. Stir one quarter of the egg whites into the ricotta mixture. Gently fold in the remaining egg whites just until blended. Pour the mixture into the crust. Sprinkle the remaining 1 tbsp crumb mixture over top. Chill for 2 hours or until the filling is set firm.

gingerbread mousse pie

Gingerbread flavour relies on molasses and ginger for its distinctive taste. It is the perfect flavour for a cookie, cake, or mousse.

CRUST
1 1/2 cups graham crumbs
1/4 cup packed brown sugar
1/4 tsp ground cinnamon
1 tbsp vegetable oil
3 tbsp water

MOUSSE
1/2 cup smooth 5% ricotta cheese
2 oz light cream cheese, softened
1/3 cup packed brown sugar
1/4 cup molasses
1/2 tsp ground cinnamon
1/4 tsp ground ginger
2 tsp unflavoured gelatin powder
3 tbsp cold water
1/2 cup low-fat yogurt
3 large egg whites
1/2 tsp cream of tartar
1/2 cup granulated sugar

MAKES 12 SERVINGS

NUTRITIONAL ANALYSIS
PER SERVING
Energy 207 calories
Protein 4.6 g
Fat, total 4.6 g
Fat, saturated 1.5 g
Carbohydrates 37 g
Fibre 0.5 g
Cholesterol 6.4 mg

NUTRITION WATCH
Molasses contains iron, calcium, and phosphorous.

TIP
Be sure when beating egg whites that the bowl and beaters are dry and clean. If the whites don't beat properly, add 1 tsp of lemon juice for every 3 egg whites and continue beating.

Spray a 9-inch pie plate with vegetable spray.

1. Make crust: In a bowl, stir together the graham crumbs, brown sugar, cinnamon, oil, and water until mixed. Set aside 1 tbsp of the crumb mixture and pat the remainder onto the bottom and up the side of a prepared pan.
2. Make mousse: In a food processor, combine ricotta cheese, cream cheese, brown sugar, molasses, cinnamon, and ginger. In a small microwavable bowl, combine the gelatin and water and let it sit for 2 minutes; microwave on high for 20 seconds. Stir the mixture until it is dissolved. With the food processor running, add the gelatin through the feed tube. Transfer it to a large bowl. Fold in the yogurt.
3. In another bowl, beat the egg whites with the cream of tartar until they are foamy. Gradually add the sugar, beating until stiff peaks form. Stir one quarter of the egg whites into the ricotta mixture. Gently fold in the remaining egg whites just until blended. Pour the mixture into the crust. Sprinkle remaining 1 tbsp over top. Chill for 2 hours or until the filling is set firm.

chocolate cream flan

NUTRITIONAL ANALYSIS
PER SERVING
Energy 288 calories
Protein 6.7 g
Fat, total 7.7 g
Fat, saturated 2.9 g
Carbohydrates 48 g
Fibre 1.2 g
Cholesterol 13 mg

NUTRITION WATCH
Condensed milk now comes
in a light version that has half
the fat of the regular version.

TIP
Light condensed milk makes
this cake smooth and rich
tasting without the addition
of egg yolks, butter, and
whipping cream.

I hope you make the sour cream spiderweb design, because it truly makes this pie exceptional looking. The filling is exceptionally delicious and so chocolatey.

CRUST
1 3/4 cups chocolate wafer
   crumbs
1 tbsp granulated sugar
1 tbsp vegetable oil
2 tbsp water

FILLING
1 can (14 oz) low-fat
   sweetened condensed milk
1/2 cup smooth 5% ricotta
   cheese
2 oz light cream cheese,
   softened
1/3 cup granulated sugar
1/4 cup unsweetened cocoa
   powder

TOPPING (OPTIONAL)
3 tbsp low-fat sour cream
1 tbsp water
2 tsp granulated sugar

Preheat the oven to 375°F. Spray a 9-inch pie plate with vegetable spray.

1. Make crust: In a bowl, mix the crumbs, sugar, oil, and water just until the crumbs come together. Pat the mixture onto side and bottom of a pie plate.
2. Make filling: In a food processor, combine the condensed milk, ricotta cheese, cream cheese, sugar, and cocoa; purée the mixture until it is smooth. Pour it into the crust.
3. Make topping: In a small bowl, stir together the sour cream, water, and sugar. Spoon the mixture into a small plastic bag and cut a tiny hole in one corner. Squeezing topping through hole, draw three concentric circles on the top of the pie. Use a toothpick to draw lines across the circles to create a spiderweb effect.
4. Place the pan in the centre of the oven and bake for 20 to 25 minutes or until the centre is firm.

apple tart

Apples and creamy cheese filling with a shortbread-type crust make a wonderful dessert. The addition of cinnamon and brown sugar to the apples brings out their flavour.

PASTRY
1/3 cup granulated sugar
3 tbsp vegetable oil
1 1/2 oz light cream cheese
1 1/4 cup all-purpose flour
3 tbsp low-fat yogurt

FILLING
1/3 cup granulated sugar
1 cup smooth 5% ricotta
  cheese
4 oz light cream cheese,
  softened
1 tsp vanilla

APPLE TOPPING
2 tsp margarine or butter
4 cups sliced, peeled apples
1/3 cup packed brown sugar
1/2 tsp ground cinnamon

Preheat the oven to 375°F. Spray a 9-inch flan pan with a removable bottom with vegetable spray.

1. Make pastry: In a food processor, purée sugar, oil, and cream cheese until the mixture is smooth. Add the flour and yogurt and process off and on until the mixture is crumbly. Roll the mixture into a bowl and wrap in plastic wrap. Chill for 20 minutes.
2. Roll the pastry between two sheets of floured wax paper into a circle large enough to fit the pan. Fit it into the pan, working the pastry up the side. Place a piece of foil over the pastry. Place in the centre of the oven and bake, covered, for 20 minutes; uncover and bake for another 10 minutes or it is until golden. Let it cool on a wire rack.
3. Make filling: In a food processor, combine sugar, ricotta cheese, cream cheese, and vanilla; purée the mixture until it is smooth. Pour it into the crust.
4. Make apple topping: In nonstick frying pan, melt the margarine over medium-high heat; cook the apples, brown sugar, and cinnamon for 5 to 7 minutes, stirring occasionally, or until apples are tender. Place the mixture on top of the filling. Chill for 1 hour.

MAKES 12 SERVINGS

NUTRITIONAL ANALYSIS
PER SERVING
Energy 228 calories
Protein 4.9 g
Fat, total 7 g
Fat, saturated 2.6 g
Carbohydrates 34 g
Fibre 1.1 g
Cholesterol 12 mg

NUTRITION WATCH
Apples are a good source of vitamins A and C.

TIP
For baking I like to use a firm sweet apple such as a Spy, Royal Gala, or Mutsu.

lime cream cheese tart

NUTRITIONAL ANALYSIS
PER SERVING
Energy 200 calories
Protein 3.3 g
Fat, total 6.0 g
Fat, saturated 2.4 g
Carbohydrates 34 g
Fibre 0.3 g
Cholesterol 33 mg

NUTRITION WATCH
Traditionally, this tart would
be made with cream cheese,
whipping cream, and heavy
14% sour cream. You can use
1% sour cream without any
loss of texture or taste.

TIPS
Buy whole vanilla wafers
and process them in the food
processor until they are
ground fine. One box contains
approximately 2 1/2 cups of
crumbs.

It takes approximately 2 to 3
limes to obtain 1/3 cup of
lime juice.

The combination of limes and a creamy cheese filling makes this tart luscious, and the vanilla wafer cookies add a buttery flavour.

CRUST
1 1/2 cups vanilla wafer
   crumbs
2 tbsp granulated sugar
2 tbsp water
1 tbsp vegetable oil

FILLING
3/4 cup granulated sugar
1 tbsp all-purpose flour
1/3 cup fresh lime juice
   (approximately 2 limes)
1 tbsp finely grated lime
   rind
3/4 cup low-fat sour cream
2 oz light cream cheese,
   softened
1 large egg
2 large egg whites

TOPPING
1 cup low-fat sour cream
3 tbsp granulated sugar

Preheat the oven to 375°F. Spray a 9-inch pie plate with vegetable spray.

1. Make crust: In a bowl, stir together the wafer crumbs, sugar, water, and oil until combined. Pat the mixture over the bottom and up the side of a prepared plate.
2. Make filling: In a food processor, purée sugar, flour, lime juice and rind, sour cream, cream cheese, egg, and egg whites until smooth. Pour it into the crust. Place the plate in the centre of the oven and bake for 25 to 30 minutes or until the centre is just set.
3. Make topping: In a bowl, stir together the sour cream and sugar. Pour the mixture carefully over the hot filling, smoothing it evenly with a knife. Return the plate to the oven and bake for 10 minutes.
4. Let the plate cool on a wire rack. Chill before serving.

orange chocolate cream cheese tart

The buttery shortbread crust, with chocolate layer and orange cream cheese filling, makes for a wonderful dessert. Top this tart with any fruit that's in season.

PASTRY
1 cup plus 2 tbsp all-purpose flour
1/3 cup granulated sugar
1/4 cup margarine or butter, cold
3 tbsp low-fat yogurt
2 tbsp water

CHOCOLATE LAYER
3 tbsp semi-sweet chocolate chips
1 tbsp water

FILLING
1/3 cup granulated sugar
1/2 cup smooth 5% ricotta cheese
2 oz light cream cheese, softened
2 tbsp orange juice concentrate
2 tsp finely grated orange rind
1/2 tsp vanilla
2 cups sliced fresh strawberries (or other fruit in season)

Preheat the oven to 375°F. Spray a 8-inch tart pan with removable bottom with vegetable spray.

1. Make pastry: In a food processor, add flour, sugar, and margarine. Pulse just until the mixture is crumbly. Add the yogurt and water and pulse just until everything is combined. Roll the dough into a ball and wrap it in plastic wrap. Chill for 20 minutes.
2. Between two floured sheets of waxed paper, roll the pastry dough into a circle large enough to fit the pan. Fit the pastry into the pan, working it up the side. Place a piece of foil over the pastry. Place the pan in the centre of the oven and bake for 10 minutes. Remove the foil and bake another 10 minutes or until the crust is golden. Let the pan cool on a wire rack.
3. Make chocolate layer: In a small microwavable bowl, combine the chocolate chips and water. Melt the chocolate chips on a high heat for approximately 30 seconds. Stir them until they are smooth. Spoon the melted chocolate over the pastry shell and use a knife to spread it thinly.
4. Make filling: In a food processor, combine sugar, ricotta cheese, cream cheese, orange juice concentrate, orange rind, and vanilla; purée the mixture until it is smooth. Pour it into the pastry shell. Top with fruit. Chill for 1 hour.

MAKES 12 SERVINGS

NUTRITIONAL ANALYSIS
PER SERVING
Energy 177 calories
Protein 3.5 g
Fat, total 6.5 g
Fat, saturated 2.2 g
Carbohydrates 26 g
Fibre 1.2 g
Cholesterol 6 mg

NUTRITION WATCH
Custard tart is usually made with a high-fat crust and a combination of egg yolks and whipping cream for the filling. The calories and fat are greatly reduced in this version.

TIP
If you want the berries to shine, melt 2 tbsp apple jelly or red currant jelly with 1 tbsp of water and brush over top.

chocolate mousse royale tart

MAKES 12 SERVINGS

NUTRITIONAL ANALYSIS
PER SERVING
Energy 182 calories
Protein 5.4 g
Fat, total 3.6 g
Fat, saturated 2.2 g
Carbohydrates 32 g
Fibre 0.8 g
Cholesterol 8.2 mg

NUTRITION WATCH
Traditional chocolate mousses
are made with egg yolks,
a lot of chocolate, and heavy
cream whipped into the
mousse. Beaten egg whites,
ricotta cheese, cocoa, and
a small amount of melted
chocolate make this a
delicious yet light-tasting
alternative.

TIP
Add the water to the chocolate to make it easier to melt
and to add moisture and
volume. Be sure to add the
melted chocolate to the
cheese mixture quickly and
process before the chocolate
begins to harden.

This was a late addition to this book! I had so many wonderful chocolate desserts that I knew one more couldn't hurt, especially a decadent mousse like this one.

MERINGUE
3 large egg whites
1/4 tsp cream of tartar
1/2 cup granulated sugar

MOUSSE
3/4 cup granulated sugar
3/4 cup smooth 5% ricotta
  cheese

2 oz light cream cheese,
  softened
1/4 cup unsweetened
  cocoa powder
3 tbsp semi-sweet
  chocolate chips
1 tbsp water
2 tsp unflavoured gelatin
  powder

3 tbsp cold water
2/3 cup low-fat yogurt
2 large egg whites
1/4 tsp cream of tartar
1/3 cup granulated sugar
Unsweetened cocoa powder
Icing sugar

Preheat the oven to 275°F. Spray a 9-inch pie plate with vegetable spray.

1. Make meringue: In a bowl, beat the egg whites with the cream of tartar until they are foamy. Gradually beat in the sugar, beating until stiff peaks form. Spoon the mixture into a prepared pan, spreading it over the bottom and up the sides. Place the pan in the centre of the oven and bake for 75 minutes or until the meringue is golden and dry. Let the pan cool on a wire rack.

2. Make mousse: In a food processor, combine 3/4 cup sugar, ricotta cheese, cream cheese, and cocoa; purée until the mixture is smooth. In a small microwavable bowl, melt the chocolate with 1 tbsp water in microwave for 40 seconds on high. Stir it until it is smooth and add it to the food processor, puréeing until the mixture is smooth.

3. In a small microwavable bowl, combine the gelatin and water and let it sit for 2 minutes; microwave on high for 20 seconds. Stir the mixture until it is dissolved. With the food processor running, add the gelatin mixture through the feed tube. Transfer the mixture to a large bowl and fold in the yogurt.

4. In another bowl, beat the egg whites with the cream of tartar until they are foamy. Gradually add 1/3 cup sugar, beating until stiff peaks form. Stir one quarter of the egg whites into the ricotta mixture. Gently fold in the remaining egg whites just until combined. Pour into the crust. Chill for 2 hours or until the filling is firm. Sprinkle cocoa and icing sugar over top.

mocha mousse chocolate chip brownie tart

When I first created this recipe, I made the crust from cookie crumbs and it tasted fine. But then I thought that a brownie base would raise this dessert to the heavens, and it does!

BROWNIE BASE
3/4 cup granulated sugar
1/4 cup vegetable oil
1/4 cup low-fat sour cream
1 large egg
1 tsp vanilla
1/3 cup all-purpose flour
1/3 cup unsweetened cocoa
  powder
1 tsp baking powder

MOUSSE
3/4 cup granulated sugar
3/4 cup smooth 5% ricotta
  cheese
2 oz light cream cheese,
  softened
2 tsp unflavoured gelatin
  powder
3 tbsp cold water
2 tsp instant coffee granules

1 tbsp hot water
2/3 cup low-fat yogurt
2 large egg whites
1/4 tsp cream of tartar
1/3 cup granulated sugar
2 tbsp semi-sweet
  chocolate chips

Preheat the oven to 350°F. Spray a 9-inch springform pan with vegetable spray.

1. Make brownie base: In a bowl and using a whisk or electric mixer, beat sugar, oil, sour cream, egg, and vanilla. In another bowl, stir together flour, cocoa, and baking powder. With a wooden spoon, stir the dry ingredients into the sugar mixture just until combined. Spread it into a prepared pan. Bake in the centre of the oven for 20 to 25 minutes or until a tester inserted in the centre comes out clean.

2. Make mousse: In a food processor, purée 3/4 cup sugar, ricotta cheese, and cream cheese until smooth. In a small bowl, stir together the gelatin and cold water; let the mixture stand for 2 minutes. Dissolve instant coffee in hot water; stir it into the gelatin mixture. Heat it in the microwave on high for 20 seconds or just until gelatin is dissolved. With the food processor running, add gelatin mixture through the feed tube. Transfer the mixture to a large bowl. Fold in the yogurt.

3. In another bowl, beat egg whites with cream of tartar until they are foamy. Gradually add 1/3 cup sugar, beating until stiff peaks form. Stir one quarter of the egg whites into the ricotta mixture. Gently fold in the remaining egg whites until blended. Pour the mixture onto the brownie base. Sprinkle with chocolate chips. Chill for 2 hours or until the filling is set firm.

MAKES 12 SERVINGS

NUTRITIONAL ANALYSIS
PER SERVING
Energy 251 calories
Protein 5.7 g
Fat, total 8 g
Fat, saturated 2.4 g
Carbohydrates 39 g
Fibre 1 g
Cholesterol 27 mg

NUTRITION WATCH
Traditional chocolate mousses are made with egg yolks, a lot of chocolate, and heavy cream. All this makes for an enormous amount of calories, fat, and cholesterol. Beaten egg whites, ricotta cheese, and cocoa in this recipe create a delicious yet light-tasting mousse.

TIP
Although most brownies are baked until they are still slightly loose in the centre, this one should be cooked through so it slices easily.

pecan shortbread tarts

These tarts are buttery and delicious. They taste like an old-fashioned butter pecan tart.

PASTRY

1/4 cup granulated sugar

2 1/2 oz light cream cheese

2 tbsp vegetable oil

1 tbsp butter

1 cup all-purpose flour

1 to 2 tbsp ice water

FILLING

3/4 cup packed brown sugar

1/4 cup corn syrup

1/3 cup toasted chopped pecans

2 tbsp evaporated skim milk

1 tbsp margarine or butter, softened

1 large egg

1 tsp vanilla

Preheat the oven to 375°F. Spray a 12-cup muffin tin with vegetable spray.

1. Make pastry: In a food processor, combine the sugar, cream cheese, oil, and butter; purée the mixture until it is smooth. Add the flour and 1 tbsp water; pulse on and off until the mixture is crumbly, adding more water as needed. Form the dough into a ball and wrap in plastic wrap. Refrigerate for 20 minutes.
2. Make filling: In a bowl, whisk together the brown sugar, corn syrup, pecans, evaporated milk, margarine, egg, and vanilla.
3. Between two sheets of floured waxed paper, roll the pastry dough out to 1/8-inch thickness. Use a 3 1/2-inch round cutter to cut out circles. Place the circles in the muffin cups, working the pastry up the side of the cups. Re-roll the pastry scraps to cut more circles. Divide the filling evenly among the pastry cups.
4. Place the tin in the centre of the oven and bake for 20 minutes or until filling is set and pastry is golden.
5. Serve the tarts warm or at room temperature.

soufflés, caramels, and brûlées

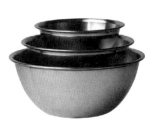

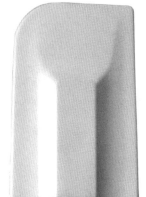

tips on divine light soufflés, caramels, and brûlées

1. A soufflé has a light and airy texture. It has a flavoured base and egg whites beaten in to increase the volume, and is baked in a water bath (bain marie) to ensure even baking and a perfect texture.

2. Crème caramel is a custard that has been baked in a caramel-coated mould. When the chilled custard is turned out onto a dish, it is already glazed and sauced with the caramel.

3. A crème brûlée is a chilled, stirred custard that is sprinkled with brown or granulated sugar. The sugar is quickly caramelized under either a broiler or torch-like instrument called a salamander. The topping becomes brittle and creates a wonderful texture and taste along with the smooth custard.

4. For creamier results use 2% milk products. The calories and fat will not differ considerably, considering these recipes make between 6 and 8 desserts.

5. The key to a perfect soufflé is beating the egg whites properly. Egg whites beat best if they are at room temperature. Always use clean and dry beaters and bowls — if there is any foreign substance in the bowl, the whites will not beat properly. Adding cream of tartar helps to stabilize the whites. Beat them until they are foamy and then gradually add the sugar while beating constantly until stiff peaks form. Fold the whites into the base mixture quickly and gently. Do not overfold or the whites will deflate.

6. Because soufflés begin to collapse in minutes, they must be served straight out of the oven. They are delicious when served with a sauce (see Sauces).

7. When making the caramel sauce for crème caramel, allow the sugar and water to boil without being stirred. It reaches the perfect consistency when the sauce is medium brown. If it cooks to the dark brown stage, the caramel will become brittle and cannot be used. If it is too light, the syrup won't caramelize and will be too runny.

8. To tell if a caramel or brûlée is ready, the centre should just appear set, not too loose and not too dry. It sets upon cooling.

chocolate soufflé

A classic soufflé is a light, airy mixture that begins with a thick egg yolk–based sauce lightened by beaten egg whites; whipped cream or rich chocolate sauce is usually added when it is served. This version has no egg yolks and is thickened with egg whites and cornstarch. Serve these heavenly delights with Chocolate Sauce (see page 240) or Crème Anglaise (see page 239).

1/2 cup granulated sugar
1/2 cup unsweetened cocoa powder
1 tbsp cornstarch
1 cup low-fat milk
6 large egg whites
1/2 tsp cream of tartar
1/2 cup granulated sugar

Preheat the oven to 350°F. Spray eight 1/2-cup ramekins with vegetable spray and dust them with sugar.

1. In a saucepan off the heat, whisk together 1/2 cup sugar, cocoa, cornstarch, and milk until smooth. Cook the mixture over medium-low heat for 4 minutes or until thickened, stirring constantly. Remove the pan from the heat. Cool.
2. In a bowl, beat the egg whites with the cream of tartar until they are foamy. Gradually add 1/2 cup sugar, beating until stiff peaks form. Stir one quarter of egg whites into the cocoa mixture. Gently fold in the remaining egg whites just until blended. Divide the mixture among the prepared ramekins.
3. Set the ramekins in a large baking dish. Pour in enough hot water to come halfway up sides of the ramekins. Bake in the centre of the oven for 20 to 25 minutes or until the soufflés are puffed. Serve them immediately.

MAKES 8 SERVINGS

NUTRITIONAL ANALYSIS
PER SERVING
Energy 153 calories
Protein 4.7 g
Fat, total 1.1 g
Fat, saturated 0.6 g
Carbohydrates 31 g
Fibre 1.8 g
Cholesterol 1.2 mg

NUTRITION WATCH
Egg whites are a complete source of protein and contain no fat. That means you can enjoy an egg-white omelette with sautéed vegetables and low-fat cheese for a nutritious breakfast.

TIPS
When whipping egg whites, take great care that the bowl and beaters are clean and dry. The egg whites will beat faster at room temperature.

For even baking, cook the soufflés in a water bath (bain marie).

orange grand marnier soufflé

NUTRITIONAL ANALYSIS
PER SERVING
Energy 144 calories
Protein 2 g
Fat, total 0 g
Fat, saturated 0 g
Carbohydrates 34 g
Fibre 0.1 g
Cholesterol 0 mg

NUTRITION WATCH
If you're going to order
dessert in a restaurant, soufflés are probably your best
choice, as long as you skip
the whipped cream and any
cream-based sauces.

TIPS
This recipe works well with
apricot or peach jam, too.

You can use an additional
2 tbsp of orange juice concentrate instead of the orange
liqueur.

The marmalade and orange juice concentrate give this soufflé an intense orange flavour.
For added flavour, serve with Mango Coulis (see page 243) or Chocolate Sauce (see page 240).

1/2 cup granulated sugar
2 tbsp cornstarch
1/2 cup water
1/4 cup orange juice concentrate
1/4 cup marmalade
2 tbsp orange-flavoured liqueur
4 large egg whites
1/4 tsp cream of tartar
1/3 cup granulated sugar

Preheat the oven to 350°F. Spray eight 1/2-cup ramekins with vegetable spray and dust them
with sugar.

1. In a saucepan off the heat, whisk together 1/2 cup sugar, cornstarch, water, orange juice concentrate, and marmalade until smooth. Cook the mixture over medium-low heat for 4 to 5 minutes
or it is until thickened, stirring constantly. Remove the pan from the heat. Stir in the liqueur.
Cool.
2. In a bowl, beat the egg whites with the cream of tartar until they are foamy. Gradually add
1/3 cup sugar, beating until stiff peaks form. Stir one quarter of the egg whites into the cooled
orange mixture. Gently fold in the remaining egg whites just until blended. Divide the mixture
among the prepared ramekins.
3. Set the ramekins in a large baking dish. Pour in enough hot water to come halfway up the sides
of the ramekins. Bake in the centre of the oven for 20 minutes or until the soufflés are puffed.
Serve them immediately.

mocha irish cream soufflé

Setting the ramekins in a pan of hot water allows the soufflés to bake evenly. This is called a bain marie or water bath. The texture results in a much creamier consistency. Serve this coffee-based soufflé with Chocolate Sauce (see page 240).

1/2 cup granulated sugar

2 tbsp cornstarch

1/2 cup low-fat milk

1 tbsp Bailey's Irish Cream or other coffee cream liqueur

1 tbsp brewed strong coffee

4 large egg whites

1/4 tsp cream of tartar

1/3 cup granulated sugar

Preheat the oven to 350°F. Spray eight 1/2-cup ramekins with vegetable spray and dust them with sugar.

1. In a saucepan off the heat, whisk together 1/2 cup sugar, cornstarch, milk, liqueur, and coffee until smooth. Cook the mixture over medium-low heat for 7 minutes or until it is thickened, stirring constantly. Remove the pan from the heat. Cool.

2. In a bowl, beat the egg whites with the cream of tartar until they are foamy. Gradually add 1/3 cup sugar, beating until stiff peaks form. Stir one quarter of the egg whites into the coffee mixture. Gently fold in the remaining egg whites just until blended. Divide among the prepared ramekins.

3. Set the ramekins in a large baking dish. Pour in enough hot water to come halfway up the sides of the ramekins. Bake in the centre of the oven for 20 minutes or until the soufflés are puffed and lightly browned. Serve them immediately.

MAKES 8 SERVINGS

NUTRITIONAL ANALYSIS
PER SERVING
Energy 110 calories
Protein 2.3 g
Fat, total 0.5 g
Fat, saturated 0.3 g
Carbohydrates 24 g
Fibre 0 g
Cholesterol 0.9 mg

NUTRITION WATCH
Low-fat milk consists of
1% MF or less. You can use
2% MF for a creamier texture.
One cup of 1% MF contains
100 calories and 2.5 g of fat,
and 2% MF contains
120 calories and 4.5 g of fat.
When you divide this among
eight servings, it doesn't
make a big difference.

TIPS
A chocolate- or coffee-based
liqueur is a wonderful addition.

If you want to omit the
alcohol, add another tablespoon of brewed coffee to the
mixture.

lemon soufflé

MAKES 6 SERVINGS

NUTRITIONAL ANALYSIS
PER SERVING
Energy 158 calories
Protein 2.4 g
Fat, total 0 g
Fat, saturated 0 g
Carbohydrates 37 g
Fibre 0.1 g
Cholesterol 0 mg

NUTRITION WATCH
Lemons are an excellent
source of vitamin C but they
begin to lose potency as soon
as they are squeezed.

TIP
Only use freshly squeezed
lemon juice. The bottled
version is not suitable for
a dessert whose flavour
depends upon lemon.

This is such a fluffy, cloud-light soufflé with a subtle lemon flavour. If you want more lemon taste, serve with Lemon Sauce (see page 243).

1/2 cup granulated sugar
1 1/2 tbsp cornstarch
1/3 cup water
2 tsp finely grated lemon rind
1/3 cup fresh lemon juice
4 large egg whites
1/4 tsp cream of tartar
1/2 cup granulated sugar

Preheat the oven to 350°F. Spray six 1/2-cup ramekins with vegetable spray and dust them with sugar.

1. In a saucepan off the heat, whisk together 1/2 cup sugar, cornstarch, water, lemon rind, and lemon juice until smooth. Cook the mixture over medium-low heat for 3 to 4 minutes or until it is thickened, stirring constantly. Remove the pan from the heat. Cool.
2. In a bowl, beat the egg whites with the cream of tartar until they are foamy. Gradually add 1/2 cup sugar, beating until stiff peaks form. Stir one quarter of the egg whites into the cooled lemon mixture. Gently fold in the remaining egg whites just until blended. Divide among the prepared ramekins.
3. Set the ramekins in a large baking dish. Pour in enough hot water to come halfway up the sides of the ramekins. Bake in the centre of the oven and for 20 to 25 minutes or until the soufflés are puffed. Serve them immediately.

crème orange caramel

A traditional crème caramel is a custard baked in a caramel-coated mould. When the chilled custard is turned out onto a serving plate, it is already glazed and sauced. In this classic dessert, the orange and caramel flavours combine well together.

CARAMEL	CUSTARD
2/3 cup granulated sugar	1 cup low-fat milk
1/3 cup water	1 cup evaporated skim milk
	3/4 cup granulated sugar
	2 large eggs
	1 large egg white
	2 tsp finely grated orange rind
	1 tsp vanilla

Preheat the oven to 350°F. Use eight ungreased 1/2-cup ramekins.

1. Make caramel: In a small saucepan, stir together 2/3 cup sugar and water. Bring the mixture to a boil, and cook for 6 to 8 minutes without stirring or until it becomes medium brown. Remove the pan from the heat. Pour the mixture into the ramekins. Pick each one up and swirl the caramel over the bottom and up the sides.
2. Make custard: In a saucepan, heat the milk with the evaporated milk.
3. In a bowl, whisk together 3/4 cup sugar, eggs, egg white, orange rind, and vanilla. Gradually whisk in the hot milk mixture. Pour the custard evenly into the ramekins.
4. Set the ramekins into a large baking dish. Pour in enough hot water to come halfway up the sides of the ramekins. Place the dish in the centre of the oven and bake 30 to 35 minutes or until the caramels are almost set.
5. Remove the ramekins from the water bath. Let them cool on a wire rack. Chill.
6. To serve, run a sharp knife around the inside edge of each ramekin and quickly invert it onto a dessert plate.

MAKES 8 SERVINGS

NUTRITIONAL ANALYSIS
PER SERVING

Energy 200 calories

Protein 5.4 g

Fat, total 1.6 g

Fat, saturated 0.6 g

Carbohydrates 41 g

Fibre 0.1 g

Cholesterol 56 mg

NUTRITION WATCH
Crème caramel is traditionally made with whipping cream, which contains 35% MF, and several egg yolks, which also contain a lot of cholesterol and fat. I have reduced the calories and fat by using low-fat milk, fewer egg yolks, and more egg whites.

TIPS
For a richer texture, use 2% milk and 2% evaporated milk.

Be sure to boil the caramel mixture just until it becomes medium brown — the glaze will be too runny if it is too light and will harden if too dark.

fudge crème custard

Cocoa, chocolate chips, and hint of chocolate liqueur make this an ultimate creamy custard.

2 cups low-fat milk
1 cup granulated sugar
1/3 cup unsweetened cocoa powder
2 large eggs
1 large egg white
1 tbsp chocolate liqueur
2 tbsp semi-sweet chocolate chips
1 tsp vanilla

Preheat the oven to 350°F. Spray eight 1/2-cup ramekins with vegetable spray.

1. In a saucepan, heat the milk.
2. In a bowl, whisk together sugar, cocoa, eggs, egg white, liqueur, chocolate chips, and vanilla. Gradually whisk in the hot milk and pour the mixture into the ramekins.
3. Set the ramekins in a large baking dish. Pour in enough hot water to come halfway up the sides of the ramekins. Bake in the centre of the oven for 30 to 35 minutes or until the custards are set.
4. Remove the ramekins from the water bath. Let them cool on a wire rack. Chill.

MAKES 8 SERVINGS

NUTRITIONAL ANALYSIS
PER SERVING
Energy 183 calories
Protein 4.9 g
Fat, total 3.5 g
Fat, saturated 1.7 g
Carbohydrates 33 g
Fibre 1.4 g
Cholesterol 56 mg

NUTRITION WATCH
Custards are traditionally
made from heavy cream and
lots of egg yolks, causing
them to be a high-fat dessert.
This recipe's use of lower fat
milk and the addition of some
egg whites and cocoa bring
the calories and fat right
down.

TIPS
You can use a creamy
chocolate liqueur, like Bailey's
Irish Cream, or a mocha or
nut-based chocolate liqueur.

If you don't want a liqueur,
add 1 tbsp chocolate syrup or
strong coffee.

mocha crème brûlée

Brûlée is the French word for "burned." The crunchy and delicious topping of this custard is set under a broiler or torch to caramelize the sugar.

1 1/2 cups low-fat milk
1/2 cup evaporated skim milk
1 tbsp instant espresso powder or instant coffee granules
2 large eggs
2 large egg whites
1/2 cup granulated sugar
3 tbsp chocolate-flavoured liqueur
2 tbsp packed brown sugar

Preheat the oven to 350°F. Use six ungreased 1/2-cup ramekins.

1. In a saucepan, heat the milk, evaporated milk, and espresso powder.
2. In a bowl, beat the eggs, egg whites, and sugar; gradually whisk in the hot milk mixture. Beat in the liqueur and pour the mixture into the ramekins.
3. Set the ramekins into a large baking dish. Pour in enough hot water to come halfway up the sides of the ramekins. Cover the dish loosely with foil. Bake 45 to 60 minutes or until the custards are set.
4. Remove the ramekins from the water bath. Let them cool on a wire rack. Chill.
5. Preheat the oven to broil. Set the top rack as close to the element as possible. Sprinkle brown sugar over the custards. Broil them until the sugar melts and caramelizes, about 1 to 2 minutes. Serve immediately.

MAKES 6 SERVINGS

NUTRITIONAL ANALYSIS
PER SERVING
Energy 174 calories
Protein 7 g
Fat, total 2.4 g
Fat, saturated 1 g
Carbohydrates 31 g
Fibre 0 g
Cholesterol 74 mg

NUTRITION WATCH
Espresso coffee actually has less caffeine than regular coffee. Espresso beans are roasted for longer, and the longer the beans roast and stronger the coffee becomes, the less the caffeine!

TIP
Instant espresso is usually available where ground coffee is sold. It is strong and gives a wonderful mocha flavour when combined with chocolate. Alternatively, use regular instant coffee — taste for flavouring and increase to 1 1/2 tbsp if necessary.

puddings, bread puddings, and pudding cakes

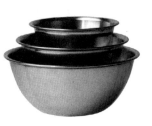

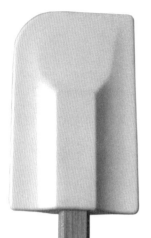

tips for divine light puddings, bread puddings, and pudding cakes

1. The secret to low-fat puddings is to use lower-fat milk, either 2% MF or less, instead of the traditional heavy cream or homogenized milk. Cornstarch and an egg thicken the puddings.

2. Combine the ingredients in the saucepan before putting it on the heat so the cornstarch dissolves. If you add the mixture to the heat before the cornstarch is dissolved, the mixture will not thicken properly and there will be lumps.

3. Use a medium-low heat so as not to burn or scald the milk. Keep whisking until the mixture begins to thicken. If an egg is called for, remove the pan from the heat before adding the egg; mix well. Return the pan to the heat and continue whisking, on a low heat, until the mixture is thickened, approximately 1 to 2 minutes.

4. Pour the pudding into individual custard cups, cover, and chill. They're best eaten the same day.

5. Bread puddings are made from cubes of bread and saturated with a mixture of milk, eggs, sugar, and flavourings. I like to use a large Italian loaf that's at least a day or two old. I remove the crusts and cut the bread into small cubes.

6. The recipes for bread puddings use lower-fat milk and fewer eggs than the traditional recipes. Their flavour is enhanced by dried fruits, coffee, cocoa, and other low-fat ingredients. These bread puddings need to be baked just until they're set and they're tastiest served warm with Crème Anglaise (see page 239) or Vanilla Cream (see page 241).

7. Pudding cakes have a texture between a cake and a pudding. Beneath the cake-like texture lies a thin layer of flavoured sauce. They're best served straight from the oven.

8. Pudding cakes are baked in a water bath (bain marie): the pan is placed in a larger pan that is filled halfway with hot water. This allows the cake to bake evenly and remain moist. The cake is set when the centre is no longer loose.

coconut rum raisin pudding

Since I discovered light coconut milk, all those recipes I never made because they were too high in fat are now possible. I'm in heaven! Coconut milk adds a silky texture and subtle flavour to desserts.

1 1/4 cups low-fat milk
1/2 cup light coconut milk
2 tbsp rum
1/2 cup granulated sugar
2 tbsp cornstarch
1 large egg
1/4 cup toasted coconut
1/4 cup raisins

Prepare six dessert dishes.

1. In a heavy-bottomed saucepan off the heat, whisk together the milk, coconut milk, rum, sugar, and cornstarch until smooth. Bring the mixture to a boil over medium-high heat, whisking constantly. Remove the pan from the heat.
2. In a bowl, whisk the egg. Whisk 1/2 cup of the hot mixture into the egg. Whisk the egg mixture back into the saucepan. Cook the mixture over medium-low heat for 1 minute, stirring, or until it is thickened and bubbling. Remove the pan from the heat.
3. Stir in the coconut and raisins. Divide the pudding among six dessert dishes, cover, and chill.

MAKES 6 SERVINGS

NUTRITIONAL ANALYSIS
PER SERVING
Energy 165 calories
Protein 3.2 g
Fat, total 4.5 g
Fat, saturated 3.4 g
Carbohydrates 28 g
Fibre 1 g
Cholesterol 37 mg

NUTRITION WATCH
Light coconut milk has 75% less fat than the regular version and is available in most grocery stores.

TIP
Instead of rum, try 2 tsp vanilla and 1 1/2 more tbsp coconut milk.

To toast coconut, heat it in a skillet on high for 1 to 2 minutes or just until it is lightly browned.

jamoca pecan pudding

One of my favourite ice creams is Jamoca Almond Fudge. This pudding is just as good.

2 cups low-fat milk
3/4 cup packed brown sugar
1/4 cup unsweetened cocoa powder
2 tbsp cornstarch
4 tsp instant coffee granules
1 large egg
3 tbsp toasted chopped pecans
2 tbsp semi-sweet chocolate chips

Prepare six dessert dishes.

1. In a heavy-bottomed saucepan off the heat, whisk together the milk, brown sugar, cocoa, corn-starch, and coffee until smooth. Bring the mixture to a boil over medium-high heat, whisking constantly. Remove the pan from the heat.
2. In a bowl, whisk the egg. Whisk 1/2 cup of the hot mixture into the egg. Whisk the egg mixture back into the saucepan. Cook the mixture over medium-low heat for 1 minute, stirring, or until it is thickened and bubbling. Remove the pan from the heat.
3. Stir in the pecans and chocolate chips. Divide the pudding among six dessert dishes, cover, and chill.

MAKES 6 SERVINGS

NUTRITIONAL ANALYSIS
PER SERVING
Energy 226 calories
Protein 5.1 g
Fat, total 5.9 g
Fat, saturated 1.9 g
Carbohydrates 38 g
Fibre 1.8 g
Cholesterol 39 mg

NUTRITION WATCH
Puddings are a great way
to increase calcium and
vitamin A, thanks to their milk
content.

TIP
To toast nuts, place in a small
skillet over high heat for
approximately 3 minutes,
until they are browned.
I often do a large batch and
freeze them for easier use.

apricot date orange pudding

The combination of dried fruits and orange makes this a tropical sweet citrus-flavoured pudding.

1 1/4 cups low-fat milk
1/2 cup evaporated skim milk
3 tbsp orange juice concentrate
1/2 cup granulated sugar
2 tbsp cornstarch
2 tsp finely grated orange rind
1 large egg
1/4 cup chopped dried apricots
1/4 cup chopped dried dates

Prepare six dessert dishes.

1. In a heavy-bottomed saucepan off the heat, whisk together the milk, evaporated milk, orange juice concentrate, sugar, cornstarch, and orange rind until smooth. Bring the mixture to a boil over medium-high heat, whisking constantly. Remove the pan from the heat.
2. In a bowl, whisk the egg. Whisk 1/2 cup of the hot mixture into the egg. Whisk the egg mixture back into saucepan. Cook the mixture over medium-low heat for 1 minute, stirring, or until it is thickened and bubbling. Remove the pan from the heat.
3. Stir in the apricots and dates. Divide the pudding among six dessert dishes, cover, and chill.

MAKES 6 SERVINGS

NUTRITIONAL ANALYSIS
PER SERVING
Energy 181 calories
Protein 4.9 g
Fat, total 1.5 g
Fat, saturated 0.6 g
Carbohydrates 37 g
Fibre 1.1 g
Cholesterol 38 mg

NUTRITION WATCH
Dried fruits are an excellent source of concentrated energy. Use them for a boost any time of day.

TIPS
I like to use orange juice concentrate due to the intensity of flavour — always keep a can in the freezer for cooking.

Store dried fruits in the freezer and use them as needed; to chop, cut them with scissors.

maple syrup walnut pudding

MAKES 6 SERVINGS

NUTRITIONAL ANALYSIS
PER SERVING
Energy 206 calories
Protein 3.8 g
Fat, total 4.8 g
Fat, saturated 1 g
Carbohydrates 37 g
Fibre 0.4 g
Cholesterol 38 mg

NUTRITION WATCH
Walnuts are a good source
of protein and are an unsaturated fat. But they contain
lots of calories and fat, so eat
them in moderation.

TIP
Be sure to buy pure maple
syrup, AA or Fancy Grade.
The imitation syrups are
nothing more than corn syrup
with maple extract.

We all know that maple syrup is good over pancakes, but try it in your baking as a substitute for honey or as an additional sweetener for heavenly results.

1 1/2 cups low-fat milk
1/2 cup maple syrup
1/3 cup packed brown sugar
3 tbsp cornstarch
1 large egg
1/4 cup chopped toasted walnuts

Prepare six dessert dishes.

1. In a heavy-bottomed saucepan off the heat, whisk together the milk, maple syrup, brown sugar, and cornstarch until smooth. Bring the mixture to a boil over medium-high heat, whisking constantly. Remove the pan from the heat.
2. In a bowl, whisk the egg. Whisk 1/2 cup of the hot mixture into the egg. Whisk the egg mixture back into the saucepan. Cook the mixture over medium-low heat for 1 minute, stirring, or until it is thickened and bubbling. Remove the pan from the heat.
3. Stir in the walnuts. Divide the pudding among six dessert dishes, cover, and chill.

chocolate cappuccino bread pudding

Bread puddings are simple, delicious, baked desserts made with cubes of bread and milk. This combination of bread, chocolate, and coffee is unique. Serve it with Chocolate Sauce (see page 240) or Crème Anglaise (see page 239).

3 cups cubed crustless day-old Italian bread
2 large eggs
1 1/3 cups evaporated skim milk
2/3 cup brewed coffee
2/3 cup granulated sugar
1/4 cup unsweetened cocoa powder
1/4 cup semi-sweet chocolate chips
1/8 tsp salt

Preheat the oven to 375°F. Spray a 8-inch square baking dish with vegetable spray.

1. Place the cubed bread in a large bowl.
2. In another bowl, whisk together the eggs, evaporated milk, coffee, sugar, cocoa, chocolate chips, and salt. Pour the mixture over the bread and cover with plastic wrap. Let it stand for 15 minutes.
3. Pour the mixture into a prepared baking dish. Bake for 30 minutes or until the pudding is set. Serve it warm.

MAKES 12 SERVINGS

NUTRITIONAL ANALYSIS
PER SERVING
Energy 144 calories
Protein 4.9 g
Fat, total 2.7 g
Fat, saturated 1.2 g
Carbohydrates 25 g
Fibre 1.2 g
Cholesterol 36 mg

NUTRITION WATCH
Evaporated milk has 60% of the water removed. It's a great substitute for cream to thicken sauces.

TIPS
Use the wide Italian bread, not the long, thin baguette, which has too much crust. Freeze any leftover bread for another use.

If brewed coffee is unavailable, dissolve 1 tbsp instant in 2/3 cup of hot water.

NUTRITIONAL ANALYSIS
PER SERVING

Energy 148 calories

Protein 3.9 g

Fat, total 1.8 g

Fat, saturated 0.6 g

Carbohydrates 29 g

Fibre 1 g

Cholesterol 37 mg

NUTRITION WATCH

If you want to save some fat
and cholesterol, replace one
of the eggs with 2 egg whites.

TIP

If you don't have buttermilk,
substitute low-fat yogurt or
make your own buttermilk by
adding 1 tbsp lemon juice to
1 cup milk and letting it sit
5 minutes.

dried fruit buttermilk bread pudding

Dried cranberries are my newest addition to baking and cooking. I replace the raisins in many
of my recipes with these tangy, chewy morsels. Dried cherries are also wonderful. Try serving
this bread pudding with Mango Coulis (see page 243).

3 cups cubed crustless day-old Italian bread

2 large eggs

2 cups buttermilk

2 tsp vanilla

3/4 cup granulated sugar

1/2 cup chopped dried apricots or dates

1/3 cup dried cranberries or raisins

1/8 tsp salt

Preheat the oven to 375°F. Spray a 8-inch square baking dish with vegetable spray.

1. Place the cubed bread in a large bowl.
2. In another bowl, whisk together the eggs, buttermilk, vanilla, sugar, apricots, cranberries, and
   salt. Pour the mixture over the bread and cover with plastic wrap. Let it stand for 15 minutes.
3. Pour the mixture into a prepared baking dish. Bake for 30 minutes or until the pudding is set.
   Serve it warm.

upside-down apple bread pudding

Upside-down cakes are so attractive, I decided to try the technique on a bread pudding. It's fabulous. Serve with Vanilla Cream (see page 241) or Crème Anglaise (see page 239).

3 1/2 cups cubed crustless day-old Italian bread

2 large eggs

1 cup low-fat milk

1 cup low-fat sour cream

2 tsp vanilla

1/2 cup packed brown sugar

1/2 tsp ground cinnamon

2 tsp margarine or butter

2 tbsp corn syrup

2 1/2 cups peeled, thinly sliced apples

3 tbsp granulated sugar

1/2 tsp ground cinnamon

Preheat the oven to 375°F. Spray a 8-inch square baking dish with vegetable spray.

1. Place the cubed bread in a large bowl.
2. In another bowl, whisk together the eggs, milk, sour cream, vanilla, brown sugar, and cinnamon. Pour the mixture over the bread and cover with plastic wrap. Let it stand for 15 minutes.
3. In a frying pan, melt the margarine with the corn syrup over medium-high heat, stirring. Stir in the apples, sugar, and cinnamon; cook for 4 minutes, stirring occasionally, or until the apples are tender. Pour the mixture into a prepared dish.
4. Pour the soaked bread on top of the apple mixture. Bake for 35 minutes or until the pudding is set. Let the dish cool slightly on a wire rack, then invert it onto a large rimmed platter. Serve it warm.

MAKES 12 SERVINGS

NUTRITIONAL ANALYSIS
PER SERVING
Energy 169 calories
Protein 3.9 g
Fat, total 3.7 g
Fat, saturated 1.7 g
Carbohydrates 30 g
Fibre 1.2 g
Cholesterol 43 mg

NUTRITION WATCH
An apple a day keeps the doctor away! Apples are a good source of vitamins A and C, as well as fibre and carbohydrates.

TIP
Choose a firm apple, like Spy or Mutsu, when baking. McIntosh and Golden Delicious lack flavour and texture when baked.

orange apricot pudding cake

Pudding cakes are best right out of the oven. They fall after they have cooled and lose their fluffy texture but are still delicious. Orange and dried apricots are a great combination in this cake.

2 large eggs, separated
3/4 cup granulated sugar
1 cup low-fat yogurt
1/4 cup apricot jam
2 tbsp orange juice concentrate
2 tsp finely grated orange rind
1/3 cup all-purpose flour
1/8 tsp salt
1/4 cup diced dried apricots
1/4 tsp cream of tartar
3 tbsp granulated sugar

Preheat the oven to 350°F. Spray a 8-inch square baking dish with vegetable spray.

1. In a large bowl and using a whisk or electric beater, beat the egg yolks with 3/4 cup sugar until the mixture is thick and pale yellow. With a wooden spoon, stir in the yogurt, jam, orange juice concentrate, orange rind, flour, salt, and apricots.
2. In another bowl and using clean beaters, beat the egg whites with the cream of tartar until they are foamy. Gradually add 3 tbsp sugar, continuing to beat until stiff peaks form. Fold the mixture into the batter just until blended. Pour it into a prepared baking dish.
3. Set the baking dish into a larger baking dish. Pour in enough hot water to reach halfway up the side of the dish. Bake for 25 to 30 minutes or until the cake is golden and the top is firm to the touch. Serve it immediately.

lemon pudding cake

Any lemon dessert makes me weak at the knees. This one has the texture of a soufflé but is slightly denser. Serve it right out of the oven, with Vanilla Cream (see page 241).

2 large eggs, separated
2/3 cup granulated sugar
1 cup low-fat yogurt
1 tbsp finely grated lemon rind
1/4 cup fresh lemon juice
1/4 cup all-purpose flour
1/4 tsp cream of tartar
3 tbsp granulated sugar

Preheat the oven to 350°F. Spray a 8-inch square baking dish with vegetable spray.

1. In a large bowl and using a whisk or electric beater, beat the egg yolks with 2/3 cup sugar until the mixture is thick and pale yellow. With a wooden spoon, stir in the yogurt, lemon rind, lemon juice, and flour.
2. In another bowl and using clean beaters, beat the egg whites with the cream of tartar until they are foamy. Gradually add 3 tbsp sugar, continuing to beat until stiff peaks form. Fold the mixture into the batter just until blended. Pour it into a prepared baking dish.
3. Set the baking dish into a larger baking dish. Pour in enough hot water to reach halfway up the side of the dish. Bake for 25 to 30 minutes or until the cake is golden and the top is firm to the touch. Serve it immediately.

MAKES 12 SERVINGS

NUTRITIONAL ANALYSIS
PER SERVING
Energy 93 calories
Protein 2.4 g
Fat, total 1.2 g
Fat, saturated 0.5 g
Carbohydrates 18 g
Fibre 0.1 g
Cholesterol 37 mg

NUTRITION WATCH
Lemons are an excellent source of vitamin C — they provide between 40% and 70% of the minimum daily requirements — but they start to lose their nutritional potency as soon as they're squeezed.

TIP
I always use fresh lemon juice, rather than bottled, when the recipe depends on lemon for its taste. Bottled lemon juice has a bitter after-taste. I often squeeze a few lemons and freeze the juice in ice cube trays for later use.

coconut cranberry pudding cake

MAKES 12 SERVINGS

NUTRITIONAL ANALYSIS
PER SERVING
Energy 115 calories
Protein 2 g
Fat, total 2.6 g
Fat, saturated 1.8 g
Carbohydrates 21 g
Fibre 0.7 g
Cholesterol 36 mg

NUTRITION WATCH
One quarter cup regular
coconut milk has 11 g of fat
and 110 calories. The light
version has 36 calories and
3 g of fat.

TIPS
Light coconut milk, now available in most grocery stores,
has 75% less fat than regular,
which is loaded with fat,
cholesterol, and calories.

The water bath (bain marie)
allows the cake to bake
evenly and retain the smooth
texture.

Dried cranberries are replacing raisins in many recipes today. They have a wonderfully tart taste that adds flavour to your baking. Light coconut milk is another great find for low-fat cooking.

2 large eggs, separated
2/3 cup granulated sugar
1/2 cup light coconut milk
1/2 cup low-fat yogurt
1/3 cup dried cranberries
1/4 cup all-purpose flour
4 tbsp toasted coconut
1 1/2 tsp vanilla
1/8 tsp salt
1/4 tsp cream of tartar
3 tbsp granulated sugar

Preheat the oven to 350°F. Spray a 8-inch square baking dish with vegetable spray.

1. In a large bowl and using a whisk or electric beater, beat the egg yolks with 2/3 cup sugar until the mixture is thick and pale yellow. With a wooden spoon, stir in the coconut milk, yogurt, cranberries, flour, 3 tbsp coconut, vanilla, and salt.
2. In another bowl and using clean beaters, beat the egg whites with the cream of tartar until they are foamy. Gradually add 3 tbsp sugar, continuing to beat until stiff peaks form. Fold the mixture into the batter just until blended. Pour it into a prepared baking dish.
3. Set the baking dish into a larger baking dish. Pour in enough hot water to reach halfway up the side of the dish. Bake for 25 to 30 minutes or until the cake is golden and the top is firm to the touch. Sprinkle with remaining 1 tbsp coconut. Serve it immediately.

four spice pudding cake

The combination of these spices and molasses makes an unbelievably tasty cake. Pudding cakes are an unusual combination of pudding and cake: you get the creaminess of a pudding and the texture of a cake.

2 large eggs, separated
1 cup packed brown sugar
3 tbsp molasses
1 cup low-fat yogurt
1/3 cup all-purpose flour
1/2 tsp ground cinnamon
1/4 tsp ground ginger
1/8 tsp allspice
1/8 tsp nutmeg
1/4 tsp cream of tartar
3 tbsp granulated sugar

Preheat the oven to 350°F. Spray a 8-inch square baking dish with vegetable spray.

1. In a large bowl and using a whisk or electric beater, combine the egg yolks, brown sugar, and molasses. With a wooden spoon, stir in the yogurt, flour, cinnamon, ginger, allspice, and nutmeg.
2. In another bowl and using clean beaters, beat the egg whites with the cream of tartar until they are foamy. Gradually add the sugar, continuing to beat until stiff peaks form. Fold the mixture into the batter just until blended and pour it into a prepared baking dish.
3. Set the baking dish into a larger baking dish. Pour in enough hot water to reach halfway up the side of the dish. Bake for 25 to 30 minutes or until the cake no longer moves when you shake the dish. Serve it immediately.

MAKES 12 SERVINGS

NUTRITIONAL ANALYSIS
PER SERVING
Energy 137 calories
Protein 2.5 g
Fat, total 1.2 g
Fat, saturated 0.5 g
Carbohydrates 29 g
Fibre 0.2 g
Cholesterol 37 mg

NUTRITION WATCH
A pudding cake is a great low-fat dessert because there is no added fat. The sauce-like texture combined with the cake texture makes a deceptively smooth, velvety taste and appearance.

TIP
You can use only two or three of the four spices, keeping in mind that allspice and nutmeg are stronger.

mocha fudge pudding cake

MAKES 12 SERVINGS

NUTRITIONAL ANALYSIS
PER SERVING
Energy 139 calories
Protein 2.7 g
Fat, total 1.8 g
Fat, saturated 0.9 g
Carbohydrates 27 g
Fibre 0.6 g
Cholesterol 36 mg

NUTRITION WATCH
Most flavoured yogurts are
available in 1% MF, which is
low in calories and cholesterol. I often use them in
baking, especially as they are
a good source of protein and
calcium.

TIP
If brewed coffee is not on
hand, substitute 1 tsp instant
coffee dissolved in 2 tbsp
hot water.

Try a flavoured yogurt to enhance this pudding such as vanilla or coffee. Coffee and chocolate are a perfect combination. Try serving it with Chocolate Sauce (see page 240).

2 large eggs, separated
1 cup granulated sugar
2 tbsp strong brewed coffee
1 cup low-fat yogurt
1/4 cup all-purpose flour
3 tbsp unsweetened cocoa powder
1/8 tsp salt
1/4 tsp cream of tartar
3 tbsp granulated sugar
2 tbsp semi-sweet chocolate chips

Preheat the oven to 350°F. Spray a 8-inch square baking dish with vegetable spray.

1. In a large bowl and using a whisk or electric beater, beat the egg yolks, 1 cup sugar, and coffee. With a wooden spoon, stir in the yogurt, flour, cocoa, and salt.

2. In another bowl and using clean beaters, beat the egg whites with the cream of tartar until they are foamy. Gradually add 3 tbsp sugar, continuing to beat until stiff peaks form. Fold the mixture into the batter just until blended. Pour it into a prepared baking dish.

3. Set the baking dish into a larger baking dish. Pour in enough hot water to reach halfway up the side of the dish. Bake for 15 minutes. Scatter chocolate chips on top. Bake 10 to 15 minutes longer or until the top is firm to the touch. Serve it immediately.

squares, bars, and brownies

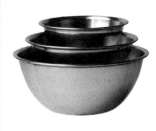

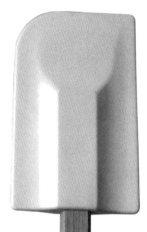

tips for divine light squares, bars, and brownies

1. Most of the recipes in this section call for an 8-inch square pan. Either glass or metal can be used. Glass will cook slightly quicker so check it 5 minutes before the baking time is done. Always spray or grease the pan well.

2. Preheat the oven and have the ingredients at room temperature before mixing.

3. Choose a whisk, hand beater, or food processor according to the filling. Be sure that the ingredients are well incorporated.

4. Cheesecake bars have a pastry crust that will be tough and dry if it is overmixed, so mix the batter just until everything is well incorporated. Pat the crust into the pan along the bottom and slightly up the sides.

5. The filling for cheesecake bars must be processed well so the batter is smooth. They are baked like a cheesecake, just until the centre is still slightly loose. Let them cool on a wire rack until they are room temperature, and then chill them before serving.

6. Oatmeal squares have a crust made of oatmeal, flour, sugar, and some oil. You don't have to worry about the mixing of these crusts — just combine the ingredients until everything comes together. Bake them until the crust is golden and crisp. If you're using dried fruit, be sure that it is pitted.

7. Brownies are simple and quick to make. Always mix the wet ingredients first and then add the dry ingredients just until they are incorporated. Do not overmix or the brownies will be dry. For the best texture, bake them just until the centre is slightly loose. Let them cool in the pan on a wire rack, and serve them right from the pan.

8. Squares, bars, and brownies can be kept at room temperature for a couple of days. They can be frozen if they are well wrapped in plastic wrap or foil, and placed in freezer bags for 6 weeks. Cheesecake bars must be refrigerated, and can also be frozen.

cheesecake shortbread squares

This shortbread cookie crust with a layer of creamy cheesecake filling is irresistible.
I like to decorate each square with a piece of fresh fruit.

CRUST
1/2 cup granulated sugar
1 large egg
1 tbsp vegetable oil
1/2 tsp vanilla
3/4 cup all-purpose flour

FILLING
1/2 cup granulated sugar
1 tbsp all-purpose flour
3/4 cup smooth 5% ricotta
    cheese
1/4 cup light cream cheese,
    softened
2 tbsp low-fat sour cream
1 large egg white
1/2 tsp vanilla

Preheat the oven to 350°F. Spray an 8-inch square cake pan with vegetable spray.

1. Make crust: In a bowl, stir together sugar, egg, oil, and vanilla. Stir in the flour until combined. Pat the crust onto the bottom and slightly up the sides of the pan.
2. Make filling: In a food processor, combine sugar, flour, ricotta cheese, cream cheese, sour cream, egg white, and vanilla; purée the mixture until it is smooth.
3. Bake in the centre of the oven for 20 to 25 minutes or until it is just slightly loose in the centre.
4. Let the pan cool on a wire rack. Serve chilled.

MAKES 16 SERVINGS

NUTRITIONAL ANALYSIS
PER SERVING
Energy 114 calories
Protein 3 g
Fat, total 2.9 g
Fat, saturated 1.2 g
Carbohydrates 19 g
Fibre 0.2 g
Cholesterol 19 mg

NUTRITION WATCH
Traditional cheesecake is
made with 35% MF cream
cheese and eggs. These
squares use a combination of
ricotta cheese and cream
cheese with egg white, so the
fat and calories are greatly
reduced.

TIP
Most shortbread crusts are
made with butter and contain
lots of calories and fat. In my
version I use only a small
amount of oil.

chocolate sour cream cheesecake squares

Chocolate cheesecake in any way, shape, or form is not to be refused. These luscious squares have a brownie type of crust that is simply mouth watering. They're so good, I featured them on the front cover!

CRUST
1/2 cup granulated sugar
3 tbsp unsweetened cocoa powder
2 tbsp vegetable oil
1 large egg
1/2 tsp vanilla
2/3 cup all-purpose flour

FILLING
2/3 cup granulated sugar
2 tbsp unsweetened cocoa powder
1 tbsp all-purpose flour
2/3 cup 5% smooth ricotta cheese
1/4 cup light cream cheese, softened
2 tbsp low-fat sour cream
1 large egg white
1/2 tsp vanilla

TOPPING
1 oz white or semi-sweet chocolate
   chunks or 2 tbsp chocolate chips

Preheat the oven to 350°F. Spray an 8-inch square baking dish with vegetable spray.

1. Make crust: In a bowl, stir together sugar, cocoa, oil, egg, and vanilla. Stir in the flour just until combined. Pat the mixture into the bottom of the dish.
2. Make filling: In a food processor, combine sugar, cocoa, flour, ricotta cheese, cream cheese, sour cream, egg white, and vanilla; purée until the mixture is smooth. Spread it over the crust. Sprinkle with chocolate.
3. Bake in the centre of the oven for 20 to 25 minutes or until the centre is still slightly loose in the middle.
4. Let the dish cool on a wire rack.

brownie cream cheese squares with sliced berries

These brownie squares with a cream cheese topping and sliced berries are downright decadent and are incredibly moist.

CAKE

2 tsp instant coffee granules

3 tbsp hot water

3/4 cup granulated sugar

3 tbsp vegetable oil

1 large egg yolk

1 tsp vanilla

1/2 cup all-purpose flour

3 tbsp unsweetened cocoa powder

1 tsp baking powder

2 large egg whites

1/4 tsp cream of tartar

3 tbsp granulated sugar

TOPPING

2/3 cup smooth 5% ricotta cheese

1 1/2 oz light cream cheese, softened

1/3 cup icing sugar

1 1/2 tsp water

1/2 tsp vanilla

1 cup sliced strawberries

Preheat the oven to 350°F. Spray a 9-inch square metal cake pan with vegetable spray.

1. In large bowl, dissolve the instant coffee in hot water. With a whisk or electric beater, add 3/4 cup sugar, oil, egg yolk, and vanilla; mix until everything is combined.

2. In another bowl, stir together the flour, cocoa, and baking powder. With a wooden spoon, stir the mixture into the coffee mixture until combined.

3. In separate bowl and using clean beaters, beat the egg whites with the cream of tartar until they are foamy. Gradually add 3 tbsp sugar, beating until stiff peaks form. Fold the egg whites into the batter just until blended. Pour the mixture into a prepared dish.

4. Bake in the centre of the oven for 20 to 25 minutes, just until the centre is just set. Let the dish cool on a wire rack.

5. Make topping: In a food processor, combine ricotta cheese, cream cheese, icing sugar, water, and vanilla; purée until the mixture is smooth. Spread the mixture over the cake. Arrange the strawberries over top.

MAKES 16 SERVINGS

NUTRITIONAL ANALYSIS PER SERVING

Energy 127 calories

Protein 2.8 g

Fat, total 4.4 g

Fat, saturated 1.2 g

Carbohydrates 19 g

Fibre 0.7 g

Cholesterol 18 mg

NUTRITION WATCH

The sliced berries on top of these brownies provide an excellent source of vitamin C and also provide some potassium and iron.

TIP

The trick to perfect brownies is to underbake them slightly, so the centre is just a little loose. Overbaking them makes them dry.

orange chocolate squares with cream cheese icing

MAKES 16 SERVINGS

NUTRITIONAL ANALYSIS
PER SERVING
Energy 127 calories
Protein 1.8 g
Fat, total 3.7 g
Fat, saturated 0.8 g
Carbohydrates 21 g
Fibre 0.6 g
Cholesterol 15 mg

NUTRITION WATCH
Icings are usually made with
butter, lard, or vegetable
shortening. Using a little light
cream cheese makes them
lower in fat, calories, and
cholesterol and they're delicious with any cake.

TIPS
Keep a container of frozen
orange juice in the freezer to
use only for cooking and baking purposes.

Store-bought chocolate sauce
is usually made from sugar,
corn syrup, and cocoa. There
usually is no fat, but if you're
not certain try the Chocolate
Sauce on page 240.

Orange and chocolate have always been a wonderful combination. The orange juice concentrate is what gives this cake its intense orange flavour.

CAKE
3/4 cup granulated sugar
2 tsp finely grated orange rind
1/4 cup orange juice concentrate
3 tbsp Chocolate Sauce (see page 240)
   or store-bought chocolate sauce
3 tbsp vegetable oil
1 large egg
1/4 cup low-fat yogurt
3/4 cup all-purpose flour
3 tbsp unsweetened cocoa powder
1 tsp baking powder
1/2 tsp baking soda

ICING
2 oz light cream cheese, softened
1/2 cup icing sugar
1 tbsp orange juice concentrate

Preheat the oven to 350°F. Spray an 8-inch square baking dish with vegetable spray.

1. Make cake: In a bowl and using a whisk or electric mixer, beat sugar, orange rind, orange juice concentrate, chocolate sauce, oil, egg, and yogurt.
2. In another bowl, stir together flour, cocoa, baking powder, and baking soda. With a wooden spoon, stir the mixture into the orange mixture until mixed. Spread it into a prepared dish.
3. Bake in the centre of the oven for 25 to 30 minutes or until a tester inserted into the centre comes out dry.
4. Let the dish cool on a wire rack.
5. Make icing: In a food processor, combine cream cheese, icing sugar, and orange juice concentrate; purée until the mixture is smooth. Spread it over the cake.

date pecan oatmeal squares

Date squares, often known as matrimonial squares, have been a classic for decades. The oatmeal crust often contains a cup or more of butter or vegetable shortening. My version only uses 1/3 cup oil mixed with some water, and it's incredibly delicious and rich tasting.

1 1/2 cups (8 oz) chopped pitted dates
1/4 cup granulated sugar
1 cup orange juice
1 1/4 cups quick-cooking oats
1 cup all-purpose flour
3/4 cup packed brown sugar
1/4 cup chopped toasted pecans
1/2 tsp ground cinnamon
1/3 cup vegetable oil
1/4 cup water

Preheat the oven to 350°F. Spray an 8-inch square baking dish with vegetable spray.

1. In a saucepan, combine the dates, sugar, and orange juice. Bring the mixture to a boil and then simmer over medium heat for 15 minutes or until dates are soft and liquid is absorbed. Mash the mixture and let it cool.
2. In a bowl, stir together oats, flour, brown sugar, pecans, cinnamon, oil, and water until combined. Pat half of the mixture onto the bottom of a prepared dish. Spread the date mixture over top. Sprinkle the remaining oat mixture on top of the dates.
3. Bake in the centre of the oven for 25 minutes or until the squares are golden.
4. Let the dish cool on a wire rack.

NUTRITIONAL ANALYSIS
PER SERVING
Energy 211 calories
Protein 2.4 g
Fat, total 6.4 g
Fat, saturated 0.5 g
Carbohydrates 36 g
Fibre 2.1 g
Cholesterol 0

NUTRITION WATCH
Dates are an excellent source of energy and carbohydrates, as well as protein and iron. Eat them in moderation, because their nutrients and calories are concentrated.

TIPS
I buy my pitted dates at a bulk food store and keep them in the freezer.

To chop dried fruits, I use scissors, which is easier than a knife.

Toast pecans in a skillet over a high heat until they are lightly browned.

apricot oatmeal squares

In my original cookbook on light cooking, *Rose Reisman Brings Home Light Cooking*, I had a traditional yet low-fat version of date squares. I still make them but this version calls for apricots instead of dates. They're great.

PURÉE	CRUST
8 oz dried apricots	1 cup quick-cooking oats
1/4 cup granulated sugar	3/4 cup all-purpose flour
1 cup water	2/3 cup packed brown sugar
	1/2 cup Grape-Nuts cereal
	1/2 tsp baking powder
	1/2 tsp baking soda
	1/2 tsp ground cinnamon
	1/3 cup vegetable oil
	3 tbsp water

Preheat the oven to 350°F. Spray an 8-inch baking dish with vegetable spray.

1. Make purée: In a saucepan, combine apricots, sugar, and water. Bring the mixture to a boil; reduce the heat to medium-low and simmer for 15 to 20 minutes, uncovered, or until the apricots are very soft. Transfer the mixture to a food processor and purée.
2. Make crust: In a bowl, stir together oats, flour, brown sugar, cereal, baking powder, baking soda, cinnamon, oil, and water until crumbly. Divide the mixture in half. Pat one half into the bottom of a prepared dish. Spread the apricot purée on top. Sprinkle the crust mixture over top.
3. Bake in the centre of the oven for 20 minutes or until the squares are golden. Let the dish cool on a wire rack.

orange cranberry squares

Dried cranberries and orange go well together in these squares. You can always use another dried fruit of your choice, such as dried cherries, raisins, dates, or apricots, too.

SQUARES
1/3 cup packed brown sugar
1/3 cup granulated sugar
2 tsp finely grated orange rind
1/4 cup fresh orange juice
3 tbsp vegetable oil
1 large egg
1 tsp vanilla
1 cup all-purpose flour
1/2 cup dried cranberries
1/2 tsp baking powder
1/2 tsp ground cinnamon

TOPPING
1 tbsp granulated sugar
1/8 tsp ground cinnamon

Preheat the oven to 350°F. Spray an 8-inch square baking dish with vegetable spray.

1. Make squares: In a bowl and using a whisk or electric mixer, beat brown sugar, sugar, orange rind, orange juice, oil, egg, and vanilla.
2. In another bowl, stir together flour, cranberries, baking powder, and cinnamon. With a wooden spoon, stir the mixture into the orange mixture until mixed. Spread into a prepared dish.
3. Make topping: In a small bowl, stir together sugar and cinnamon. Sprinkle the mixture over the squares.
4. Bake in the centre of the oven for 15 to 20 minutes or until a tester inserted into the centre comes out dry.
5. Let the dish cool on a wire rack.

MAKES 12 SERVINGS

NUTRITIONAL ANALYSIS
PER SERVING
Energy 143 calories
Protein 1.7 g
Fat, total 4 g
Fat, saturated 0.4 g
Carbohydrates 25 g
Fibre 0.8 g
Cholesterol 18 mg

NUTRITION WATCH
Dried cranberries are very high in vitamin C and can be a high-energy snack any time. You only need a small amount since their nutrients and calories are concentrated.

TIP
These squares freeze well. I like to include them in my children's lunch boxes. In fact, I like them as an afternoon snack, too, when I'm picking up the kids!

cinnamon pumpkin oatmeal squares

MAKES 16 SERVINGS

NUTRITIONAL ANALYSIS
PER SERVING
Energy 146 calories
Protein 1.9 g
Fat, total 4 g
Fat, saturated 0.4 g
Carbohydrates 25 g
Fibre 1.3 g
Cholesterol 13.5 mg

NUTRITION WATCH
These squares are loaded
with nutrition. Pumpkin is a
good source of vitamin A,
oats are high in vitamin B1,
and dates are a good source
of protein and iron.

TIP
Don't buy pumpkin pie filling,
which contains sugar and
other ingredients. Buy pure,
puréed pumpkin, with nothing
added.

The pumpkin, oatmeal, and dates make these squares chewy and moist. Great for a lunch-time snack or a breakfast nibble.

1 cup packed brown sugar
1/2 cup canned pumpkin purée
1/3 cup low-fat milk
1/4 cup vegetable oil
1 large egg
1 tsp vanilla
3/4 cup all-purpose flour
2/3 cup quick-cooking oats
1/2 cup chopped pitted dates or raisins
1 tsp baking powder
1 tsp ground cinnamon
1/4 tsp ground ginger
1/8 tsp allspice

Preheat the oven to 350°F. Spray an 8-inch square baking dish with vegetable spray.

1. In a bowl and using a whisk or electric mixer, beat brown sugar, pumpkin, milk, oil, egg, and vanilla.
2. In another bowl, stir together flour, oats, dates, baking powder, cinnamon, ginger, and allspice. With a wooden spoon, stir the mixture into the pumpkin mixture just until everything is combined. Pour the batter into a prepared dish.
3. Bake in the centre of the oven for 25 to 30 minutes or until a tester inserted into the centre comes out dry.
4. Let the dish cool on a wire rack.

maple syrup dried cherry oatmeal bars

These bars are a great snack for mid-day or in your little angels' school lunches. The maple syrup and oatmeal give the bars a chewy, moist texture.

1/2 cup packed brown sugar

1/3 cup maple syrup

1 large egg

3 tbsp vegetable oil

1 1/2 tsp vanilla

3/4 cup quick-cooking oats

2/3 cup all-purpose flour

1/3 cup dried cherries

1 tsp baking powder

Preheat the oven to 350°F. Spray an 8-inch square baking dish with vegetable spray.

1. In a bowl and using a whisk or electric mixer, beat the brown sugar, maple syrup, egg, oil, and vanilla.
2. In another bowl, stir together the oats, flour, cherries, and baking powder. With a wooden spoon, stir the mixture into the maple mixture until combined. Spread it into the prepared dish.
3. Bake in the centre of the oven for 15 to 18 minutes or until a tester inserted into the centre comes out dry.
4. Let the dish cool on a wire rack.

MAKES 12 SERVINGS

NUTRITIONAL ANALYSIS PER SERVING

Energy 150 calories

Protein 2.1 g

Fat, total 4.2 g

Fat, saturated 0.4 g

Carbohydrates 26 g

Fibre 0.9 g

Cholesterol 18 mg

NUTRITION WATCH

Rolled oats are high in vitamin B1 and contain a good amount of vitamins B2 and E.

TIP

Always buy pure maple syrup for the best flavour. The imitation brands are mostly corn syrup with the addition of artificial maple extract.

molasses oatmeal bars

NUTRITIONAL ANALYSIS
PER SERVING
Energy 141 calories
Protein 1.9 g
Fat, total 4.1 g
Fat, saturated 0.4 g
Carbohydrates 24 g
Fibre 0.6 g
Cholesterol 18 mg

NUTRITION WATCH
Molasses contains iron,
calcium, and phosphorous.

TIPS
When buying rolled oats, use
either regular old fashioned
or quick-cooking. Avoid the
instant because it gives a
sticky texture to your baking.

Molasses comes from the
process of refining sugar cane
and sugar beets. The juice is
squeezed from the plants and
boiled into a syrupy mixture.
Each subsequent boiling
produces light, dark, then
blackstrap molasses. For baking, dark is the best choice.

Molasses, oatmeal, and gingerbread spices make a wonderful-tasting bar. It's my version of a granola bar.

1/2 cup packed brown sugar
1/2 tsp ground cinnamon
1/4 tsp ground ginger
1/8 tsp allspice
1/3 cup molasses
3 tbsp vegetable oil
1 large egg
3/4 cup all-purpose flour
1/2 cup quick-cooking oats
1 tsp baking powder

Preheat the oven to 350°F. Spray an 8-inch square baking dish with vegetable spray.

1. In a bowl and using a whisk or electric mixer, beat brown sugar, cinnamon, ginger, allspice, molasses, oil, and egg.
2. In another bowl, stir together flour, oats, and baking powder. With a wooden spoon, stir the mixture into the molasses mixture until blended. Spread it into a prepared dish.
3. Bake in the centre of the oven for 15 to 18 minutes or until a tester inserted into the centre comes out dry.
4. Let the dish cool on a wire rack.

chewy peanut oatmeal bars

The peanut butter, oatmeal, and peanut butter chips make this an outstanding bar for a quick snack. I pack them in the kids' lunches and offer them as an after-school treat.

1/2 cup packed brown sugar
1/2 cup granulated sugar
1/4 cup smooth peanut butter
1/4 cup low-fat milk
2 tbsp vegetable oil
1 large egg
1 tsp vanilla
3/4 cup all-purpose flour
2/3 cup quick-cooking oats
3 tbsp peanut butter chips or semi-sweet
    chocolate chips
1/2 tsp baking soda

Preheat the oven to 350°F. Spray an 8-inch square baking dish with vegetable spray.

1. In a bowl and using a whisk or electric mixer, beat brown sugar, sugar, peanut butter, milk, oil, egg, and vanilla.
2. In another bowl, stir together flour, oats, peanut butter chips, and baking soda. With a wooden spoon, stir the mixture into the peanut butter mixture until everything is well combined. Pat it into a prepared dish.
3. Bake in the centre of the oven for 25 minutes or until a tester inserted into the centre comes out dry.
4. Let the dish cool on a wire rack.

MAKES 16 SERVINGS

NUTRITIONAL ANALYSIS
PER SERVING
Energy 144 calories
Protein 3 g
Fat, total 4.8 g
Fat, saturated 0.7 g
Carbohydrates 21 g
Fibre 0.9 g
Cholesterol 13 mg

NUTRITION WATCH
Oatmeal is still a great way to start your day. This food is classified as a low-glycemic food, which means that it raises your blood sugar slowly (this keeps you full longer).

TIP
Peanut butter chips are available in most grocery stores. You can also use semi-sweet chocolate chips or, for a different flavour altogether, try mint-flavoured chocolate chips.

pumpkin cream cheese bars

MAKES 16 SERVINGS

NUTRITIONAL ANALYSIS
PER SERVING
Energy 177 calories
Protein 3.1 g
Fat, total 4.6 g
Fat, saturated 1.1 g
Carbohydrates 30 g
Fibre 0.5 g
Cholesterol 18 mg

NUTRITION WATCH
Pumpkin is a good source of
vitamin A. Any fruit purée is a
great way to reduce the fat in
a recipe because it gives
moisture and texture to your
baking.

TIPS
Make sure you buy pure
puréed pumpkin, and not
pumpkin pie filling.

Freeze any leftover purée for
a later use.

I love pumpkin pie and I love cheesecake. Since I can't have both at once, I decided to create this unusual and delicious recipe. The combination is great.

BASE	CHEESECAKE LAYER
3/4 cup packed brown sugar	1/2 cup smooth 5% ricotta cheese
1/4 cup granulated sugar	2 oz light cream cheese, softened
1/2 tsp ground cinnamon	1/3 cup granulated sugar
1/4 tsp ground ginger	1 large egg white
1/3 cup canned pumpkin purée	1/2 tsp vanilla
3 tbsp vegetable oil	
1 large egg	TOPPING
2 tbsp low-fat yogurt	1/3 cup packed brown sugar
1 cup all-purpose flour	1/4 cup all-purpose flour
1 tsp baking powder	1/2 tsp ground cinnamon
	2 tsp water
	1 1/2 tsp vegetable oil

Preheat the oven to 350°F. Spray an 8-inch square baking dish with vegetable spray.

1. Make base: In a bowl and using a whisk or electric mixer, beat brown sugar, sugar, cinnamon, ginger, pumpkin, oil, egg, yogurt, and egg.
2. In another bowl, stir together flour and baking powder. With a wooden spoon, stir the mixture into the pumpkin mixture until combined. Pour it into a prepared dish.
3. Make cheesecake layer: In a food processor, combine ricotta cheese, cream cheese, sugar, egg white, and vanilla; purée until the mixture is smooth. Pour it over the base.
4. Make topping: In a bowl, stir together brown sugar, flour, cinnamon, water, and oil until combined. Sprinkle it over the cheesecake.
5. Bake in the centre of the oven for 30 to 35 minutes or until the centre has just set and a tester inserted into the pumpkin filling comes out dry.
6. Let the dish cool on a wire rack. Chill for 2 hours. Serve at room temperature or chilled.

orange poppyseed cheesecake bars

This crust tastes like a moist shortbread cookie crust, even though it has less fat than regular shortbread. Because it is not baked, the crust stays moist. The orange-flavoured cheesecake filling is thick and creamy.

CRUST
1/2 cup granulated sugar
1 tbsp margarine or butter
1 large egg
1 tbsp orange juice concentrate
1 tsp finely grated orange rind
3/4 cup all-purpose flour

FILLING
1/2 cup granulated sugar
1 tbsp all-purpose flour
1 tsp poppyseeds
1 tsp finely grated orange rind
3/4 cup smooth 5% ricotta cheese
1/4 cup light cream cheese, softened
1 large egg white
1 tbsp orange juice concentrate

Preheat the oven to 350°F. Spray an 8-inch square baking dish with vegetable spray.

1. Make crust: In a bowl, combine sugar, margarine, egg, orange juice concentrate, and orange rind. Mix in the flour until combined. Pat the mixture into the bottom of a prepared dish. Bake in the centre of the oven for 10 minutes.
2. Make filling: In a food processor, combine sugar, flour, poppyseeds, orange rind, ricotta cheese, cream cheese, egg white, and orange juice concentrate; purée until the mixture is smooth. Pour it over the crust. Bake in the centre of the oven for 20 minutes or until the centre is slightly loose.
3. Let the dish cool on a wire rack. Chill it for at least 1 hour.

MAKES 16 SERVINGS

NUTRITIONAL ANALYSIS
PER SERVING
Energy 114 calories
Protein 3 g
Fat, total 2.7 g
Fat, saturated 1.2 g
Carbohydrates 19 g
Fibre 0.2 g
Cholesterol 26 mg

NUTRITION WATCH
Oranges are a great nutritious snack during the day. They are an excellent source of vitamin C and contain some vitamin A.

TIP
When grating rind, be careful not to grate the white pith underneath the skin. It is bitter and will ruin your dessert.

pear raisin streusel bars

The crust is a tender yet crisp base for this tasty fruit-based bar. It requires little fat because of the added water.

CRUST
3/4 cup all-purpose flour
2/3 cup quick-cooking oats
1/3 cup granulated sugar
3/4 tsp ground cinnamon
3 tbsp vegetable oil
3 tbsp water

FILLING
2 (2 cups) diced peeled pears
1/3 cup raisins
2 tbsp granulated sugar
1 tbsp fresh lemon juice

TOPPING
1/3 cup packed brown sugar
1/3 cup all-purpose flour
1/2 tsp ground cinnamon
1 tbsp margarine or butter
2 tsp water

Preheat the oven to 350°F. Spray an 8-inch square baking dish with vegetable spray.

1. Make crust: In a bowl, stir together flour, oats, sugar, cinnamon, oil, and water until combined. Pat the mixture into a prepared dish. Bake in the centre of the oven for 10 minutes.
2. Make filling: In a bowl, stir together pears, raisins, sugar, and lemon juice. Spread the mixture over the crust.
3. Make topping: In a bowl, stir together brown sugar, flour, cinnamon, margarine, and water. Sprinkle the mixture over the filling. Bake for 25 minutes or until the pears are tender.
4. Let the dish cool on a wire rack.

peanut butter and chocolate chip granola bars

Peanut butter and chocolate made a delicious combination. These granola bars are better and healthier than any commercial ones. They make a great lunch snack for the kids.

1 1/4 cups quick-cooking oats
1/2 cup packed brown sugar
1/4 cup unsweetened toasted coconut
2 tbsp semi-sweet chocolate chips
2 tbsp peanut butter chips
3 tbsp corn syrup
2 tbsp liquid honey
3 tbsp smooth peanut butter
3 tbsp vegetable oil
3 tbsp water
2 tsp vanilla

Preheat the oven to 350°F. Spray a 8-inch square cake pan with vegetable spray.

1. In large bowl, stir together oats, brown sugar, coconut, chocolate chips, peanut butter chips, corn syrup, honey, peanut butter, oil, water, and vanilla until combined. Pat the mixture into a prepared pan.
2. Bake in the centre of the oven for 20 to 25 minutes or until the top is golden and the bars seem firm.
3. Let the pan cool on a wire rack.

MAKES 16 SERVINGS

NUTRITIONAL ANALYSIS
PER SERVING
Energy 134 calories
Protein 2.1 g
Fat, total 6 g
Fat, saturated 1.6 g
Carbohydrates 18 g
Fibre 1.3 g
Cholesterol 0

NUTRITION WATCH
Using coconut to highlight a recipe is fine nutritionally, but remember it is high in calories and saturated fat, so use it sparingly.

TIPS
Always choose natural peanut butter. The commercial brands are loaded with icing sugar (as much as one third!) and are often hydrogenated, which makes them a saturated fat.

Toast the coconut in a non-stick skillet on a high heat, just until it is lightly browned, to give the flavour more intensity.

chewy cocoa granola bars

By adding some cocoa to these granola bars I created a delicious chocolate version of this popular snack. They have a chewy and moist texture.

2/3 cup packed brown sugar
2 tbsp corn syrup
2 tbsp vegetable oil
1 large egg
1 tsp vanilla
3/4 cup low-fat granola
1/2 cup all-purpose flour
3 tbsp semi-sweet chocolate chips
2 tbsp unsweetened cocoa powder
1/2 tsp baking powder

Preheat the oven to 350°F. Spray an 8-inch square baking dish with vegetable spray.

1. In large bowl with whisk or electric mixer, beat brown sugar, corn syrup, oil, egg, and vanilla.
2. In another bowl, stir together granola, flour, chocolate chips, cocoa, and baking powder. With a wooden spoon, stir the mixture into the brown sugar mixture until combined. Spread the mixture into a prepared dish.
3. Bake in the centre of the oven for 20 to 25 minutes or until the bars have set.
4. Let the dish cool on a wire rack.

MAKES 12 SERVINGS

NUTRITIONAL ANALYSIS
PER SERVING
Energy 142 calories
Protein 1.8 g
Fat, total 3.9 g
Fat, saturated 0.9 g
Carbohydrates 25 g
Fibre 0.9 g
Cholesterol 18 mg

NUTRITION WATCH
Regular granola has approximately double the fat and calories of the low-fat brands, thanks to the addition of sugar and oil. Also, beware of commercial granola bars — these are usually not a healthy low-fat snack. The homemade version is always the best choice.

TIP
Be sure to buy low-fat granola, not the regular granola, which is loaded with fat that is often hydrogenated — which causes it to become saturated.

cream cheese–filled brownies

These brownies were featured in *Rose Reisman's Light Vegetarian Cooking*, and were rated the number-one brownie recipe. The layer of cream cheese combined with the chocolate brownies makes them simply decadent.

FILLING

4 oz light cream cheese, softened

2 tbsp granulated sugar

2 tbsp low-fat milk

1 tsp vanilla extract

CAKE

1 cup packed brown sugar

1/3 cup low-fat sour cream

1/4 cup vegetable oil

1 large egg

1 large egg white

3/4 cup all-purpose flour

1/2 cup unsweetened cocoa powder

1 tsp baking powder

Preheat the oven to 350°F. Spray an 8-inch square baking dish with vegetable spray.

1. Make filling: In a food processor or bowl with an electric mixer, beat together the cream cheese, sugar, milk, and vanilla until the mixture is smooth. Set it aside.

2. Make the cake: In a large bowl, whisk together brown sugar, sour cream, oil, whole egg, and egg white. In a separate bowl, stir together flour, cocoa, and baking powder. Add the liquid ingredients to the dry ingredients, blending just until everything is mixed.

3. Pour half the cake batter into a prepared dish. Spoon the filling on top; spread it with a wet knife. Pour the remaining batter into the pan. Bake for 20 to 25 minutes or until it is just barely loose in the centre.

MAKES 16 SERVINGS

NUTRITION ANALYSIS
PER SERVING

Energy 133 calories

Protein 3 g

Fat, total 5 g

Fat, saturated 2 g

Carbohydrates 20 g

Fibre 1 g

Cholesterol 19 mg

NUTRITION WATCH

Brownies are traditionally extremely high in calories and fat because they usually contain a lot of butter or other shortening, eggs, and often sour cream. These ones are much lower in fat and calories because the cocoa replaces the high-fat chocolate.

TIPS

Double the recipe and bake it in a 9-inch square baking dish for 10 minutes longer or until it is slightly loose in the centre.

When pouring the batter, don't worry if there's a swirling pattern — the result will be attractive.

NUTRITIONAL ANALYSIS
PER SERVING
Energy 127 calories
Protein 1.8 g
Fat, total 5 g
Fat, saturated 0.6 g
Carbohydrates 18 g
Fibre 1.3 g
Cholesterol 13.5 mg

NUTRITION WATCH
Bananas are high in carbohydrates, potassium, and
vitamin C — a great nutritious low-fat snack when
you're running out the door.

TIP
To enhance the flavour of
bananas in your baking, toss
overripe ones in the freezer,
then thaw and use. The
flavour is much more intense.

chocolate banana pecan brownies

Brownies already are tops in my family. By adding bananas, I gave a whole new twist on this classic dessert. The bananas give moisture and texture.

3/4 cup granulated sugar
2 medium (2/3 cup) mashed ripe banana
3 tbsp vegetable oil
1 large egg
1 tsp vanilla
1 cup all-purpose flour
1/3 cup unsweetened cocoa powder
1/3 cup chopped pecans
1 tsp baking powder
1/3 cup low-fat yogurt

Preheat the oven to 350°F. Spray an 8-inch square baking dish with vegetable spray.

1. In a bowl and using a whisk or electric mixer, beat the sugar, banana, oil, egg, and vanilla.
2. In another bowl, stir together flour, cocoa, pecans, baking powder, and yogurt. With a wooden spoon, stir the mixture into the banana mixture just until everything is moistened. Pour the batter into a prepared pan.
3. Bake in the centre of the oven for 25 to 30 minutes or until a tester inserted in the centre comes out with just a few crumbs clinging to it. Do not overbake.
4. Let the dish cool on a wire rack.

rocky mountain brownies

When I first discovered a recipe for low-fat brownies, my whole family said they loved me forever! Now I've taken my next most favourite flavour — Rocky Mountain — and added it to this already delicious recipe.

1 cup granulated sugar
1/3 cup unsweetened cocoa powder
1/3 cup unsweetened applesauce
1/4 cup vegetable oil
1 large egg
1 tsp vanilla
1/4 cup low-fat yogurt
3/4 cup all-purpose flour
1/2 tsp baking powder
3/4 cup miniature marshmallows
1/4 cup semi-sweet chocolate chips

Preheat the oven to 350°F. Spray an 8-inch square baking dish with vegetable spray.

1. In a bowl and using a whisk or electric mixer, beat sugar, cocoa, applesauce, oil, egg, vanilla, and yogurt.
2. In another bowl, stir together flour and baking powder. Stir the mixture into the applesauce mixture just until everything is combined. Pour the batter into a prepared dish.
3. Bake in the centre of the oven for 20 minutes. Sprinkle with marshmallows and chocolate chips. Bake another 10 minutes.
4. Let the dish cool on a wire rack.

MAKES 16 SERVINGS

NUTRITIONAL ANALYSIS
PER SERVING
Energy 136 calories
Protein 1.2 g
Fat, total 5.2 g
Fat, saturated 0.9 g
Carbohydrates 22 g
Fibre 0.8 g
Cholesterol 13.5 mg

NUTRITION WATCH
Be sure to buy unsweetened applesauce. Sugar is added to some brands, which adds unnecessarily to the calories.

TIP
The addition of applesauce adds volume without fat to these brownies. Using any puréed fruit, such as bananas, cooked dates, or prunes, will do the same.

mint chocolate cream cheese brownies

MAKES 16 SERVINGS

NUTRITIONAL ANALYSIS
PER SERVING
Energy 123 calories
Protein 2.1 g
Fat, total 4.7 g
Fat, saturated 1.3 g
Carbohydrates 18 g
Fibre 0.9 g
Cholesterol 15 mg

NUTRITION WATCH
Yogurt is now available in
1% MF or less, including the
fruit-flavoured varieties.
I avoid the artificially sweetened ones. In fact, some-
times I use a plain yogurt and
add fruit and a little honey to
sweeten it.

TIP
Be careful when using mint
extract. It's quite intense, so
if you use too much you'll ruin
your baked goods.

Brownies with a cream cheese swirl and a mint flavour are so unusual. I may never go back to regular brownies again.

BROWNIES
3/4 cup granulated sugar
3 tbsp vegetable oil
1 large egg
1/2 tsp peppermint extract
1/2 cup low-fat yogurt
2/3 cup all-purpose flour
1/3 cup unsweetened cocoa powder
1 tsp baking powder
1/4 cup mint chocolate chips

CREAM CHEESE MIXTURE
2 oz light cream cheese
4 tsp granulated sugar
1 tbsp water

Preheat the oven to 350°F. Spray an 8-inch square baking dish with vegetable spray.

1. Make brownies: In a bowl, whisk together sugar, oil, egg, peppermint extract, and yogurt.
2. In another bowl, stir together flour, cocoa, baking powder, and chocolate chips. Stir the mixture into the sugar mixture just until everything is combined. Pour it into a prepared dish.
3. Make cream cheese mixture: In a food processor or using an electric hand beater, combine cream cheese, sugar, and water; purée until the mixture is smooth. Pour the mixture over top the brownie batter. Using a butter knife, swirl the cream cheese mixture through the batter.
4. Bake in the centre of the oven for 20 to 25 minutes or until the centre is slightly loose.
5. Let the dish cool on a wire rack.

peanut butter chip brownies

Chocolate and peanut butter are a natural combination. This brownie recipe, with its morsels of peanut butter chips, hits the spot.

3/4 cup granulated sugar
1/4 cup smooth peanut butter
2 tbsp vegetable oil
1 large egg
1 tsp vanilla
2/3 cup low-fat yogurt
2/3 cup all-purpose flour
1/3 cup unsweetened cocoa powder
1 tsp baking powder
1/4 cup peanut butter chips

Preheat the oven to 350°F. Spray an 8-inch square baking dish with vegetable spray.

1. In a bowl and using a whisk or electric mixer, beat together sugar, peanut butter, oil, egg, vanilla, and yogurt.
2. In another bowl, stir together flour, cocoa, baking powder, and peanut butter chips. With a wooden spoon, stir the mixture into the peanut butter mixture just until everything is combined. Pour the batter into a prepared dish.
3. Bake in the centre of the oven for 25 minutes or until a tester inserted in the centre comes out with a few crumbs attached to it.
4. Let the dish cool on a wire rack.

MAKES 16 SERVINGS

NUTRITIONAL ANALYSIS
Energy 141 calories
Protein 3.1 g
Fat, total 5.1 g
Fat, saturated 1 g
Carbohydrates 17 g
Fibre 1.2 g
Cholesterol 13.5 mg

NUTRITION WATCH
Peanut butter contains a fair amount of iron and niacin and is a source of protein. It has 100 calories and 8 g of fat per tbsp, but the fat is mono-unsaturated, which is better for you. Eat it in moderation.

TIP
Always buy pure, natural peanut butter. The commercial brands are often loaded with icing sugar, and can also be hydrogenated, turning peanut butter into a saturated fat.

soy sweets

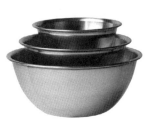

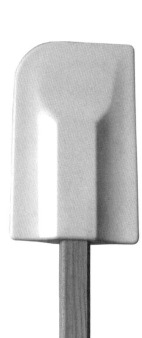

tips for divine light soy desserts

1. Soy and tofu desserts are perfect for those who are lactose intolerant, those who want to increase the soy in their diet, and those who are vegetarian and do not eat any animal products. It is also good for kosher dietary reasons, specifically no mixing meat with dairy.

2. Soy is easy to digest, is low in calories, cholesterol, and sodium, and is high in protein. It can be a source of calcium when coagulated with calcium chloride or calcium sulphate. Some can be higher in fat, so check the particular brand, although they are still lower in fat than regular sour cream or cream cheese.

3. Soy milk is the liquid squeezed from soaked soy beans. It is rich in protein and iron, cholesterol free, lactose free, and low in saturated fat. It comes in three flavours: plain, vanilla, or chocolate. Always check the fat content because certain soy products can contain higher amounts of fat than others. I use soy milk wherever I would use milk.

4. Tofu, also called soybean curd, is the vegetarian equivalent of cottage cheese in the dairy world. It can be soft, firm, or extra firm. For baking, I usually use firm to fill jelly-roll–type cakes. Be sure to process it well. Silken tofu is made from extra thick soy milk and is strained through silk, hence the name. The result is a creamy custard-like consistency, ideal for cheesecakes because it purées well.

5. Tofu can be kept, in water, in the refrigerator for up to 1 week.

6. I add salt and lots of flavouring to soy recipes because soy on its own has a bland, flat flavour and tends to absorb flavours from foods. The salt allows the other flavours to emerge.

7. You can freeze tofu if wrapped tightly for up to 6 months. The texture will change slightly but will still be fine for desserts.

lemon cheesecake

The texture of lemon and silken tofu provides a creamy texture. This cheesecake is refreshing after a heavy meal. Serve it with Raspberry Coulis (see page 242).

CRUST	FILLING
1 1/2 cups graham crumbs	1 lb soft silken tofu, drained
2 tsp granulated sugar	1/3 cup light soy milk
2 tbsp water	1 large egg
1 tbsp vegetable oil	1 cup granulated sugar
	1 tbsp finely grated lemon rind
	1/4 cup fresh lemon juice
	3 tbsp all-purpose flour
	1/4 tsp salt

Preheat the oven to 350°F. Spray a 9-inch springform pan with vegetable spray.

1. Make crust: In a bowl, stir together graham crumbs, sugar, water, and oil until combined. Pat onto the bottom and up the side of a prepared pan.
2. Make filling: In a food processor, combine tofu, soy milk, egg, sugar, lemon rind and juice, flour, and salt; purée the mixture until it is smooth. Pour it into crust.
3. Place a pan of hot water on the bottom rack of the oven. Bake the cheesecake in the centre of the oven for 45 minutes or until it is just slightly loose at the centre.
4. Run a butter knife around the edge of the cake. Let the pan cool on a wire rack until the cake is room temperature. Chill.

MAKES 12 SERVINGS

NUTRITIONAL ANALYSIS
PER SERVING
Energy 181 calories
Protein 3.8 g
Fat, total 4.2 g
Fat, saturated 0.6 g
Carbohydrates 32 g
Fibre 0.6 g
Cholesterol 18 mg

NUTRITION WATCH
Tofu is an excellent source of protein, and it is a good source of calcium when coagulated with calcium chloride or calcium sulphate.

TIP
Be sure to buy silken, not firm, tofu. Only silken will give the creamy texture this cheesecake requires.

banana marble coffee cake

MAKES 12 SERVINGS

NUTRITIONAL ANALYSIS
PER SERVING

Energy 175 calories

Protein 2.9 g

Fat, total 5.7 g

Fat, saturated 0.7 g

Carbohydrates 28 g

Fibre 1 g

Cholesterol 36 mg

NUTRITION WATCH

Soy milk comes in different
levels of milk fat. I like to use
the low-fat variety.

TIP

Be sure to keep overripe
bananas in the freezer to get
the most intense flavour. Just
defrost and mash them.

I featured this "anytime-of-day" cake in my first cookbook on light cooking, *Rose Reisman Brings Home Light Cooking.* The use of soy milk now makes it available to anyone.

1 1/3 cup all-purpose flour

1 tsp baking powder

1/2 tsp baking soda

1/4 tsp salt

2 ripe (2/3 cup, mashed) small bananas

3/4 cup light soy milk

2 large eggs

1/4 cup vegetable oil

1 tsp vanilla

1 cup granulated sugar

2 tbsp granulated sugar

1 tbsp unsweetened cocoa powder

Preheat the oven to 350°F. Spray a 9-inch square baking dish with vegetable spray.

1. In a bowl, stir together flour, baking powder, baking soda, and salt.
2. In a food processor, combine bananas, soy milk, eggs, oil, vanilla, and 1 cup sugar; purée the mixture until it is smooth. Pour it over the dry ingredients; with a wooden spoon, stir until everything is combined. Set aside 1/3 cup of the batter. Pour the remaining batter into a prepared baking dish.
3. Stir 2 tbsp sugar and cocoa into the reserved batter. Drizzle the mixture over the top of the cake batter. Using a butter knife, swirl the dark batter into the light batter.
4. Bake in the centre of the oven for 35 to 40 minutes or until a tester inserted in the centre comes out clean.
5. Let the pan cool on a wire rack.

glazed mocha cake

This cake was such a hit in my first light cookbook, *Rose Reisman Brings Home Light Cooking*, that I have adapted it to soy milk.

CAKE
1 tbsp instant coffee granules
1/3 cup hot water
3/4 cup granulated sugar
1/4 cup vegetable oil
2 large eggs
1/4 cup unsweetened cocoa powder
1 cup all-purpose flour
1 tsp baking powder
1 tsp baking soda
1/8 tsp salt
1/2 cup light soy milk

GLAZE
2/3 cup icing sugar
1 tsp instant coffee granules
1 1/2 tbsp hot water

Preheat the oven to 350°F. Spray a 9-inch springform pan with vegetable spray.

1. Dissolve the instant coffee in hot water.
2. In a bowl and using a whisk or electric beater, beat together sugar, oil, and eggs. Add the cocoa and beat until everything is blended.
3. In another bowl, stir together flour, baking powder, baking soda, and salt. Pour the cocoa mixture, soy milk, and coffee over the dry ingredients; with a wooden spoon, stir just until everything is combined. Pour the mixture into a prepared pan.
4. Bake for 30 to 35 minutes or until a tester inserted in the centre comes out clean. Let the pan cool on a wire rack. Remove the springform side.
5. Make glaze: Dissolve the instant coffee in hot water. In small bowl, mix the icing sugar with the coffee until the mixture is smooth. Spread it over the top of the cake, smoothing with a knife.

MAKES 12 SERVINGS

NUTRITIONAL ANALYSIS
PER SERVING
Energy 180 calories
Protein 2.9 g
Fat, total 5.8 g
Fat, saturated 0.8 g
Carbohydrates 29 g
Fibre 1 g
Cholesterol 35 mg

NUTRITION WATCH
Normally, icings for cakes are made from butter, cream cheese, or vegetable oil, which are all loaded with fat, calories, and cholesterol. This icing is free of fat and cholesterol.

TIP
For a real coffee zing, try using 1/3 cup strong brewed coffee or espresso instead of instant coffee.

banana chocolate meringue pie

MAKES 12 SERVINGS

NUTRITIONAL ANALYSIS
PER SERVING

Energy 237 calories

Protein 3.8 g

Fat, total 5.7 g

Fat, saturated 1.4 g

Carbohydrates 42 g

Fibre 1.8 g

Cholesterol 35 mg

NUTRITION WATCH

Bananas are high in carbohydrates and low in fat.
They're rich in potassium and
vitamin C. I love them as an
energizing snack.

TIP

Using salt is necessary when
using soy products because
the soy seems to prevent the
taste of other foods from
coming through. Salt
enhances those flavours.

This was another classic dessert from *Rose Reisman's Light Vegetarian Cooking.* The soy milk makes this delicious and caters to those who are lactose intolerant.

CRUST
1 1/2 cups chocolate wafer
   crumbs
2 tbsp water
1 tbsp vegetable oil

FILLING
1 1/3 cups light soy milk
3/4 cup granulated sugar
3 tbsp unsweetened cocoa
   powder
2 tbsp cornstarch
1/8 tsp salt
2 large egg yolks
3 tbsp semi-sweet chocolate
   chips
1 tsp vanilla
2 ripe medium bananas

MERINGUE TOPPING
3 large egg whites
1/4 tsp cream of tartar
1/2 cup granulated sugar

Preheat the oven to 425°F. Spray a 9-inch springform pan with vegetable spray.

1. Make crust: In a bowl, stir together wafer crumbs, water, and oil until mixed. Pat the mixture onto the bottom and up the side of a prepared pan. Let it chill while you make the filling.
2. Make filling: In a saucepan, heat 2/3 cup soy milk until it is hot. In a bowl, whisk the remaining soy milk, sugar, cocoa, cornstarch, salt, and egg yolks until they are smooth. Whisk the hot soy milk into the bowl. Return the mixture to the saucepan and cook it over medium heat, whisking, for 4 minutes or until thickened. Remove it from the heat. Stir in the chocolate chips and vanilla until the chips melt. Slice the bananas and arrange them over the bottom of the crust. Pour the hot filling over top.
3. Make meringue topping: In a bowl, beat the egg whites with the cream of tartar until they are foamy. Gradually add the sugar, beating until stiff peaks form. Spoon the mixture over the hot filling, spreading it to the sides of the pan.
4. Bake in the centre of the oven for 8 to 10 minutes or until the pie is golden. Let the pan cool on a wire rack.

sour cream apple pie

The cooked apples with the puréed flavoured tofu and crunchy topping make this an exceptional dessert.

CRUST
1 1/2 cups graham wafer
   crumbs
2 tbsp packed brown sugar
3 tbsp water
1 tbsp vegetable oil

FILLING
4 cups sliced peeled apples
1/2 cup granulated sugar
1/4 cup raisins
3 tbsp all-purpose flour
1 tsp ground cinnamon
3/4 cup silken tofu,
   drained
1 large egg, beaten
1 tsp vanilla

TOPPING
1/3 cup packed brown sugar
1/4 cup all-purpose flour
1/4 cup quick-cooking oats
1/2 tsp ground cinnamon
2 tsp vegetable oil
1 tsp water

Preheat the oven to 350°F. Spray a 9-inch springform pan with vegetable spray.

1. Make crust: In a bowl, stir together graham crumbs, brown sugar, water, and oil until mixed. Pat the mixture onto the bottom and up the side of a prepared pan.
2. Make filling: In a bowl, stir together the apples, sugar, raisins, flour, and cinnamon.
3. With a food processor, purée the tofu, egg, and vanilla. Add to the apple mixture and pour it into the crust.
4. Make topping: In a small bowl, stir together the brown sugar, flour, oats, cinnamon, oil, and water until crumbly. Sprinkle it over the filling.
5. Bake in the centre of the oven for 30 minutes or until the topping is golden and apples are tender.
6. Let the pan cool on a wire rack.

MAKES 16 SERVINGS

NUTRITIONAL ANALYSIS
PER SERVING
Energy 164 calories
Protein 2.4 g
Fat, total 3.4 g
Fat, saturated 0.4 g
Carbohydrates 31 g
Fibre 1.3 g
Cholesterol 13 mg

NUTRITION WATCH
Apples are a good source of vitamins A and C. They are a good source of carbohydrates and fibre, and make a great energizing snack.

TIP
I like to use a delicious-tasting apple for this dessert. My preferences are Mutsu, Royal Gala, or Spy. I avoid the Golden Delicious and the McIntosh, which I think are too soft and not as flavourful in baking.

creamy orange tart

The texture of the silken tofu is perfect for this creamy orange tart. Be sure to process the mixture well.

NUTRITIONAL ANALYSIS
PER SERVING
Energy 215 calories
Protein 2.5 g
Fat, total 5 g
Fat, saturated 0.8 g
Carbohydrates 40 g
Fibre 0.4 g
Cholesterol 1.4 mg

NUTRITION WATCH
A good way to introduce soy
in your diet if you don't like
regular tofu is to try desserts
made with it. You can replace
ricotta cheese or cream
cheese with silken tofu.

TIP
Vanilla wafers usually come
as whole cookies in a box.
I place the wafers in the food
processor and purée until
they are finely ground.
One box is approximately
2 1/2 cups of ground crumbs.

CRUST
1 1/2 cups vanilla wafer crumbs
1 tbsp granulated sugar
2 tbsp water
1 tbsp vegetable oil

FILLING
8 oz silken tofu, drained
3/4 cup light soy milk
1 1/4 cups granulated sugar
3 tbsp cornstarch
1/4 tsp salt
1/4 cup orange juice concentrate
2 tsp finely grated orange rind
Grated orange rind

Preheat the oven to 350°F. Spray a 9-inch flan pan with removable bottom with vegetable spray.

1. Make crust: In a bowl, stir together the wafer crumbs, sugar, water, and oil until combined. Pat the mixture onto the bottom and up the side of a prepared pan.
2. Make filling: In a food processor, combine tofu, sugar, cornstarch, salt, orange juice concentrate, and orange rind; purée the mixture until it is smooth. Pour it into the crust.
3. Bake in the centre of the oven for 25 to 30 minutes or until the filling is set.
4. Let the pan cool on a wire rack. Garnish with grated orange rind and chill for at least 2 hours.

bailey's irish cream chocolate pudding

After a filling meal, I enjoy a light flavourful pudding. This one does the trick.

1/4 cup unsweetened cocoa powder
3/4 cup packed brown sugar
2 1/2 tbsp cornstarch
2 tsp instant coffee granules
2 cups light soy milk
1 large egg
1 tbsp Bailey's Irish Cream liqueur
2 tbsp semi-sweet chocolate chips

Spray eight 1/2-cup ramekins with vegetable spray and dust them with sugar.

1. In a saucepan off the heat, whisk in cocoa, brown sugar, cornstarch, instant coffee, and soy milk until the mixture is smooth. Bring it to a boil over medium-high heat, whisking constantly. Remove the pan from the heat.
2. In a bowl, whisk the egg. Whisk 1/2 cup hot mixture into the egg. Whisk the egg mixture back into the saucepan. Cook over medium-low heat for 1 minute, stirring, or until the mixture is thickened and bubbling. Remove the pan from the heat. Stir in the liqueur. Divide the pudding among eight dessert dishes and chill.
3. Serve sprinkled with chocolate chips.

MAKES 8 SERVINGS

NUTRITIONAL ANALYSIS PER SERVING

Energy 158 calories
Protein 3.7 g
Fat, total 2.6 g
Fat, saturated 1.1 g
Carbohydrates 30 g
Fibre 1.6 g
Cholesterol 27 mg

NUTRITION WATCH
Soy milk is rich in protein and iron. It is cholesterol free and lactose free.

TIPS
If you don't have Bailey's Irish Cream, use another chocolate or coffee liqueur. Even a chocolate syrup will work.

I've tried this recipe with chocolate and vanilla soy milk, and it is delicious.

peanut butter pudding

Puddings are a real comfort food. The use of soy milk makes this available to anyone. The use of peanut butter and chips is decadent.

3/4 cup granulated sugar

3 tbsp cornstarch

2 cups light soy milk

1/4 cup smooth peanut butter

2 tbsp peanut butter chips

1. In a saucepan off the heat, whisk together the sugar, cornstarch, and soy milk until the mixture is smooth. Whisk in the peanut butter. Bring the mixture to a boil over medium-high heat, whisking constantly. Reduce the heat to medium-low and simmer for 4 minutes, whisking occasionally, or until the mixture is thickened and smooth.
2. Divide the mixture among six dessert dishes, cover, and chill.
3. Serve sprinkled with chips.

MAKES 8 SERVINGS

NUTRITIONAL ANALYSIS
PER SERVING

Energy 179 calories

Protein 4.5 g

Fat, total 5.2 g

Fat, saturated 0.9 g

Carbohydrates 28 g

Fibre 1.2 g

Cholesterol 0

NUTRITION WATCH

Peanut butter is high in calories and fat, but keep in mind it's rich in protein and the fat is monounsaturated, which has been known to lower the bad cholesterol in your blood. But eat it in moderation.

TIP

Always buy natural peanut butter, which only contains peanuts. Commercial brands contain icing sugar, and are often hydrogenated, making them a form of saturated fat.

chocolate rice pudding

When I first served this pudding to my family, no one guessed there was soy milk in it. The texture is light and creamy and the flavour is intensely rich.

3 2/3 cups light soy milk
1 cup packed brown sugar
1/2 cup arborio rice
1/4 cup unsweetened cocoa powder
2 tbsp semi-sweet chocolate chips

1. In a heavy-bottomed medium saucepan, combine the soy milk, brown sugar, rice, and cocoa. Bring the mixture to a simmer over medium heat, stirring often. Reduce the heat to low; cook, partially covered and stirring occasionally, for 50 minutes or until the rice is tender and the mixture is thickened.
2. Remove the pan from the heat. Let it cool slightly. Stir in the chocolate chips. Pour into six dessert dishes. Serve the pudding warm or at room temperature.

MAKES 8 SERVINGS

NUTRITIONAL ANALYSIS PER SERVING
Energy 235 calories
Protein 5.5 g
Fat, total 2 g
Fat, saturated 0.8 g
Carbohydrates 48 g
Fibre 2.2 g
Cholesterol 0

NUTRITION WATCH
Rice is gluten free and an excellent source of complex carbohydrates.

TIP
Arborio rice, a high-starch Italian rice, is shorter and fatter than any other short grain rice. It's traditionally used in risotto, but is great in rice puddings.

rice pudding with dates and apricots

MAKES 8 SERVINGS

NUTRITIONAL ANALYSIS
PER SERVING

Energy 180 calories

Protein 5.4 g

Fat, total 0.5 g

Fat, saturated 0.1 g

Carbohydrates 37 g

Fibre 2.1 g

Cholesterol 0

NUTRITION WATCH

Dried fruits, such as apricots
and dates, are a wonderful,
quick source of energy, carbohydrates, and fibre. But be
careful: because they are
dried, they are concentrated
and higher in calories.

TIP

I like arborio rice, which is the
short grain rice traditionally
used in risottos. You can also
use medium grain rice. Brown
rice provides more fibre, but
you need to increase the soy
milk to 4 or 4 1/2 cups and
cook 15 minutes longer, or
until the rice is tender.

This is a sure way to get my children to have soy in their diet, especially since they don't love tofu. No one will know the difference.

3 3/4 cups light soy milk
1/2 cup arborio rice
1/3 cup granulated sugar
1/2 tsp ground cinnamon
1 tsp vanilla
1/3 cup chopped dried apricots
1/3 cup chopped dried dates

1. In a heavy-bottomed saucepan, combine soy milk, rice, sugar, and cinnamon. Bring the mixture to a simmer over medium heat, stirring often. Reduce the heat to medium-low; cook, partially covered and stirring occasionally, for 45 to 50 minutes or until the rice is tender and the mixture is thickened.
2. Stir in the vanilla, apricots, and dates. Serve it warm or at room temperature.

apple cinnamon noodle pudding cake

I featured this recipe using dairy products in *Sensationally Light Pasta and Grains*. The substitution of silken tofu makes a wonderful and creamy pudding cake.

PUDDING

8 oz wide egg noodles

1 lb silken tofu, drained

1 large egg

1 large egg white

1 tbsp finely grated orange rind

1/4 cup fresh orange juice

3/4 cup granulated sugar

1/2 tsp ground cinnamon

1/4 tsp salt

1/8 tsp nutmeg

1 cup sliced peeled apples

1/3 cup raisins or dried cranberries

1 tbsp granulated sugar

1/2 tsp ground cinnamon

TOPPING

1/3 cup packed brown sugar

1/4 cup all-purpose flour

3 tbsp quick-cooking oats

2 tsp margarine or butter

1/4 tsp ground cinnamon

Preheat the oven to 350°F. Spray a 9-inch springform pan with vegetable spray.

1. In a large pot of boiling water, cook the noodles for 8 minutes or until they are tender but firm. Drain. Rinse them under cold running water; drain.
2. In a food processor, combine the tofu, egg, egg white, orange rind and juice, 3/4 cup sugar, 1/2 tsp cinnamon, salt, and nutmeg; purée the mixture until it is smooth.
3. In a large bowl, stir together the apples, raisins, 1 tbsp sugar, and 1/2 tsp cinnamon. Stir in the tofu mixture and noodles. Pour everything into a prepared pan.
4. Make topping: In a small bowl, stir together brown sugar, flour, oats, margarine, and cinnamon until crumbly. Sprinkle the mixture over noodle mixture.
5. Bake in the centre of the oven for 35 minutes or until it is set. Either serve it warm, at room temperature, or chilled.

MAKES 12 SERVINGS

NUTRITIONAL ANALYSIS PER SERVING

Energy 220 calories

Protein 6 g

Fat, total 3.1 g

Fat, saturated 0.6 g

Carbohydrates 42 g

Fibre 1.3 g

Cholesterol 36 mg

NUTRITION WATCH

Keep in mind that egg noodles contain egg yolks, thus making them slightly higher in fat and cholesterol. Eating them occasionally is fine.

TIP

Only use egg noodles for this dessert. They differ from regular pasta because they contain eggs or egg yolks. I use the dried version and cook them according to the package directions.

mocha brownies with creamy icing

These brownies are wonderfully moist and delicious, with the addition of soy milk.

MAKES 16 SERVINGS

NUTRITIONAL ANALYSIS
PER SERVING
Energy 108 calories
Protein 1.5 g
Fat, total 3.3 g
Fat, saturated 0.5 g
Carbohydrates 18 g
Fibre 1 g
Cholesterol 13 mg

NUTRITION WATCH
Light soy milk is slightly higher in protein than cow's milk.
It's a non-dairy product rich in
iron, and it's cholesterol free
and low in fat and sodium.

TIP
If you don't have instant
coffee, use 1 1/2 tbsp brewed
strong coffee.

BROWNIES
2 tsp instant coffee granules
1 tbsp hot water
3 tbsp vegetable oil
1 large egg
3/4 cup granulated sugar
1/2 cup all-purpose flour
1/3 cup unsweetened cocoa powder
1 tsp baking powder
1/3 cup light soy milk

ICING
1/2 cup icing sugar
2 tbsp unsweetened cocoa powder
1 1/2 tbsp light soy milk

Preheat the oven to 350°F. Spray a 9-inch square cake pan with vegetable spray.

1. Make brownies: In a large bowl, dissolve instant coffee in hot water. Add oil, egg, and sugar; using a whisk or electric mixer, beat until the mixture is smooth.
2. In another bowl, stir together flour, cocoa, and baking powder. Add the dry ingredients to the coffee mixture alternately with the soy milk, in two batches, stirring with a wooden spoon just until everything is blended. Pour the mixture into a prepared baking pan.
3. Bake for 18 to 20 minutes or until the edges begin to pull away from the pan (the centre will still be slightly soft). Let the pan cool on a wire rack.
4. Make icing: In a small bowl, beat together the icing sugar, cocoa, and soy milk until the mixture is smooth. Spread it over the brownies.

chocolate coffee tiramisu

I developed a wonderful chocolate tiramisu in *Enlightened Home Cooking*, which used ricotta cheese and beaten egg whites. I find this tofu version has its own character and is delicious.

1 lb firm tofu, drained
3/4 cup granulated sugar
3 tbsp unsweetened cocoa powder
1 large egg yolk
1 tsp vanilla
1/8 tsp salt
3 large egg whites
1/4 tsp cream of tartar
1/2 cup granulated sugar
1/2 cup brewed strong coffee
1 tbsp chocolate liqueur
20 3-inch ladyfinger cookies

Use an ungreased 9-inch square baking dish.

1. In a food processor, combine tofu, 3/4 cup sugar, cocoa, egg yolk, vanilla, and salt; purée the mixture until it is smooth. Transfer it to a large bowl.
2. In another bowl, beat the egg whites with the cream of tartar until they are foamy. Gradually add 1/2 cup sugar, beating until stiff peaks form. Stir one quarter of the egg whites into the tofu mixture. Gently fold in the remaining egg whites just until blended.
3. In a small bowl, stir together the coffee and liqueur. One at a time, dip half of each ladyfinger in the mixture and place it in the bottom of the baking dish. Pour the remaining cocoa-tofu mixture over the ladyfingers. Repeat layers. Chill for at least 3 hours.

MAKES 16 SERVINGS

NUTRITIONAL ANALYSIS
PER SERVING
Energy 180 calories
Protein 7.2 g
Fat, total 4.4 g
Fat, saturated 1.1 g
Carbohydrates 27 g
Fibre 1.1 g
Cholesterol 73 mg

NUTRITION WATCH
Firm tofu is an excellent source of protein, and contains no cholesterol.

TIPS
If you don't have brewed coffee on hand, dissolve 1 tbsp instant coffee dissolved in 1/2 cup hot water.

Ladyfingers come in all sizes and in either a hard or soft texture. Either will work. If using large ones, you need only 10 to 12, and you can break them to fit the pan.

apricot roll

This apricot- and orange-flavoured roll is light and delicious with a creamy apricot filling. Serve it with Mango Coulis (see page 243).

(see page 243)

FILLING
8 oz firm tofu, drained
1/2 cup granulated sugar
1/3 cup apricot jam
1 tsp finely grated
    orange rind
1 tsp vanilla
1/8 tsp salt

2 tbsp icing sugar
1/3 cup diced dried apricots

CAKE
1 large egg
1/3 cup granulated sugar
2 tsp finely grated
    orange rind

1/4 cup fresh orange juice
2/3 cup all-purpose flour
1/2 tsp baking powder
3 large egg whites
1/4 tsp cream of tartar
1/4 cup granulated sugar
Icing sugar

Preheat the oven to 350°F. Line a 15-inch × 10-inch jelly roll pan with parchment paper and spray it with vegetable spray.

1. Make filling: In a food processor, combine tofu, sugar, jam, orange rind, vanilla, and salt; purée the mixture until it is smooth. Chill it while you make the cake.
2. Make cake: In a bowl and using a whisk or electric mixer, beat egg with 1/3 cup sugar until the mixture is thickened and pale yellow. Beat in the orange rind and juice.
3. In a separate bowl, sift the flour with the baking powder; gently fold the mixture into the egg mixture.
4. In another bowl and using clean beaters, beat the egg whites with the cream of tartar until they are foamy. Gradually beat in 1/4 cup sugar, beating until stiff peaks form. Stir one quarter of egg whites into the cake batter. Gently fold in the remaining egg whites just until blended. Spread the mixture into a prepared pan.
5. Bake in the centre of the oven for 12 minutes or until a tester comes out dry.
6. Let the pan cool on a wire rack.
7. Dust the cake with icing sugar. Invert it onto a clean tea towel. Remove the pan and peel off parchment paper. Spread the filling over the surface. Sprinkle it with apricots. Starting from the short end, gently roll up the cake with the help of the tea towel. Transfer the roll to a serving platter, seam side down. Sprinkle it with extra icing sugar to garnish.

MAKES 8 SERVINGS

NUTRITIONAL ANALYSIS PER SERVING
Energy 269 calories
Protein 8 g
Fat, total 3.2 g
Fat, saturated 0.6 g
Carbohydrates 52 g
Fibre 1.4 g
Cholesterol 27 mg

NUTRITION WATCH
Dried apricots are rich in vitamin A, and are a valuable source of iron, calcium, potassium, and fibre.

TIPS
Buy dried apricots in a bulk food store and keep them in the freezer.

Use scissors to cut dried fruit into pieces.

mocha roll

This coffee-flavoured roll is moist and delicious, without added fat, and the tofu filling is creamy and smooth. Serve it with Chocolate Sauce (see page 240).

CAKE

2 large egg yolks

1/3 cup granulated sugar

3 tbsp brewed strong coffee

1/3 cup all-purpose flour

1/4 cup unsweetened cocoa powder

4 large egg whites

1/4 tsp cream of tartar

1/2 cup granulated sugar

FILLING

8 oz firm tofu, drained

1/2 cup granulated sugar

2 tbsp unsweetened cocoa powder

1 tbsp brewed strong coffee

1/8 tsp salt

2 tbsp icing sugar

Icing sugar

Preheat the oven to 350°F. Line a 15-inch × 10-inch jelly roll pan with parchment paper and spray it with vegetable spray.

1. Make cake: In a bowl and using a whisk or electric mixer, beat the egg yolks with 1/3 cup sugar until they are thickened and pale yellow. Beat in the coffee.

2. In a separate bowl, sift the flour with the cocoa; gently fold the dry ingredients into the yolk mixture just until mixed.

3. In another bowl and using clean beaters, beat the egg whites with the cream of tartar until they are foamy. Gradually beat in 1/2 cup sugar, beating until stiff peaks form. Stir one quarter of the egg whites into the cake batter. Gently fold in the remaining egg whites just until blended. Spread the mixture into a prepared pan.

4. Bake in the centre of the oven for 15 minutes or until a tester inserted in the centre comes out clean. Let the pan cool on a wire rack.

5. Make filling: In a food processor, combine tofu, sugar, cocoa, coffee, and salt; purée the mixture until it is smooth.

6. Dust the cake with icing sugar. Invert it onto a clean tea towel. Remove the pan and peel off the parchment paper. Spread the filling over the cake. Starting from the short end, gently roll up the cake with the help of the tea towel. Sprinkle the cake with extra icing sugar to garnish.

MAKES 8 SERVINGS

NUTRITIONAL ANALYSIS PER SERVING

Energy 245 calories

Protein 8.3 g

Fat, total 4.4 g

Fat, saturated 1.1 g

Carbohydrates 43 g

Fibre 2.1 g

Cholesterol 53 mg

NUTRITION WATCH

Tofu is easy to digest, is low in calories, cholesterol, and sodium, and is high in protein. Some tofus can be higher in fat. Check the particular kind you are using.

TIPS

If brewed coffee is not on hand, dissolve 1/2 tsp instant coffee in 3 tbsp hot water.

Be sure to use firm tofu, not soft.

lemon poppyseed loaf

This was one of my most delicious desserts in my first cookbook on light cooking, *Rose Reisman Brings Home Light Cooking*. The silken tofu gives the loaf a light and creamy texture. I often make one and eat it the same day, or make a couple and freeze them.

MAKES 12 SERVINGS

NUTRITIONAL ANALYSIS
PER SERVING
Energy 166 calories
Protein 2.7 g
Fat, total 5.7 g
Fat, saturated 0.6 g
Carbohydrates 26 g
Fibre 0.5 g
Cholesterol 18 mg

NUTRITION WATCH
Lemons are an excellent
source of vitamin C, but they
lose approximately half of
their benefits as soon as
they're squeezed.

TIP
As with any dish that relies
on lemon for its taste, use
only fresh lemon juice for this
dessert.

LOAF
3/4 cup granulated sugar
3/4 cup silken tofu, drained
2 tsp finely grated lemon rind
1/4 cup fresh lemon juice
1/4 cup vegetable oil
1 large egg
1 1/4 cups all-purpose flour
2 tsp poppyseeds
1 tsp baking powder
1/2 tsp baking soda
1/4 tsp salt

GLAZE
1/4 cup icing sugar
2 tbsp fresh lemon juice

Preheat the oven to 350°F. Spray a 9-inch × 5-inch loaf pan with vegetable spray.

1. Make loaf: In a food processor, combine the sugar, tofu, lemon rind and juice, oil, and egg; purée the mixture until it is smooth. Add the flour, poppyseeds, baking powder, baking soda, and salt; pulse on and off just until everything is combined. Pour the mixture into a prepared pan.
2. Bake in the centre of the oven for 25 to 30 minutes or until a tester comes out dry.
3. Let the pan cool on a wire rack.
4. Make glaze: In a bowl, beat the icing sugar with the lemon juice until the mixture is smooth. Poke holes in the cake while it is still in the pan. Pour the glaze over the cake. Let the cake cool completely before serving.

passover desserts

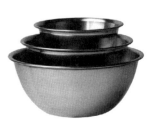

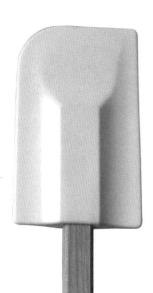

tips for divine light passover desserts

1. When you are baking for Passover, avoid wheat flour, except for matzo, and any foods containing flour, such as ladyfingers and cookie crumbs.

2. Avoid leavening agents such as yeast and baking powder.

3. Avoid cornstarch and corn syrup, which are derivatives of corn.

4. Avoid cream of tartar because it is made during alcohol distillation.

5. The following products require a Passover label: vanilla and other extracts, because regular extracts are made with grain alcohol; yogurt; powdered sugar, which must be made without cornstarch; dried fruits; matzo and matzo products; oils, of which only peanut oil is permissible; and vinegar.

6. These products require a label only if purchased during Passover: salt, which must not be iodized; spices; frozen fruits and juices; milk; butter; baking soda; nuts; cocoa; cottage cheese; coffee; sugar; and honey.

7. For chocolate, use pareve Passover chocolate or chocolate chips (pareve means acceptable for kosher use). Don't buy chocolate that does not contain cocoa butter, because it doesn't taste like chocolate and doesn't melt well.

8. Coconut products are not usually made specifically for Passover, but people who are more lenient in their dietary restrictions can include it in the recipes.

9. None of these recipes requires gelatin, but if you have a Passover recipe requiring gelatin you must use kosher gelatin. Whisk the gelatin into cold liquid and then quickly bring it to a boil. It begins to set immediately so add it to the remaining ingredients at once.

10. You can use jams or jellies — just make sure they don't contain corn syrup.

11. Matzo cake meal is a very finely ground mild-tasting product perfect for baking. But don't substitute it for matzo meal, which is just coarsely ground matzo.

12. Peanut butter is acceptable for Conservative congregations.

13. Potato starch is used in smaller quantities in baking along with matzo cake meal. The balance of both produces a better texture and taste.

14. Passover cakes do not rise as in traditional cakes. They are smaller and denser, with an intense flavour and texture.

banana layer cake with chocolate icing

Banana and chocolate are a great combination, especially with a creamy icing.

CAKE

1 cup granulated sugar

2 ripe (2/3 cup) small bananas, mashed

2 large eggs

1/3 cup vegetable oil

1 1/2 tsp vanilla

3/4 cup matzo cake meal

1/3 cup potato starch

4 large egg whites

1/2 cup granulated sugar

ICING

2 1/2 oz light cream cheese, softened

2/3 cup Passover icing sugar

3 tbsp unsweetened cocoa powder

1/3 cup low-fat sour cream

1 ripe medium banana

Preheat the oven to 350°F. Spray three 8-inch round cake pans with vegetable spray.

1. Make cake: In a large bowl and using a whisk or electric mixer, beat 1 cup icing sugar, 2 bananas, eggs, oil, and vanilla. With a wooden spoon, stir in the cake meal and potato starch until combined.
2. In another bowl, beat the egg whites until they are foamy. Gradually add 1/2 cup sugar, beating until stiff peaks form. Stir one quarter of the egg whites into the batter. Gently fold in the remaining egg whites just until combined. Divide the mixture among the prepared cake pans.
3. Bake in the centre of the oven for 15 to 20 minutes or until a tester inserted in the centre comes out clean.
4. Let the pans cool on a wire rack.
5. Make icing: In a food processor, combine cream cheese, sugar, cocoa, and sour cream; purée the mixture until it is smooth.
6. Place one cake layer on a cake platter. Spread some of the icing over top. Slice the banana; place half on the cake layer. Place the second cake layer on top of the first. Spread some of the icing over top. Place the remaining banana slices on top. Place the third cake layer on top of the second. Ice the top and sides.

NUTRITIONAL ANALYSIS
PER SERVING

Energy 284 calories

Protein 4.2 g

Fat, total 8.8 g

Fat, saturated 1.8 g

Carbohydrates 47 g

Fibre 1.3 g

Cholesterol 41 mg

NUTRITION WATCH

Bananas provide a high source of potassium, as well as some vitamin A and fibre.

TIPS

I always keep ripe bananas in the freezer so I have them on hand for baking. Nothing tastes better.

To ripen bananas, place them in a perforated brown paper bag for a few days.

chocolate layer cake with italian meringue

NUTRITION WATCH
Cocoa is chocolate without the cocoa butter, which contains the fat and cholesterol. One ounce of chocolate has 9 g of fat. One ounce of cocoa has 3 g.

TIPS
Don't confuse matzo cake meal with matzo meal. Cake meal is finer and produces a more tender cake.

The light and fluffy meringue topping is delicious on other cakes, too.

Passover desserts are usually terribly high in fat and calories, due to the excessive use of eggs and oil. Not this one! I adore this cake all year round, but it's a special treat at Passover, with its fluffy and creamy meringue topping.

CAKE
2 large egg yolks
2/3 cup granulated sugar
1/3 cup vegetable oil
2/3 cup low-fat yogurt
1/3 cup unsweetened
  cocoa powder

1/3 cup matzo cake meal
2 tbsp potato starch
4 large egg whites
1/3 cup granulated sugar

ICING
3 large egg whites
3/4 cup granulated sugar
1/4 cup water
2 tbsp unsweetened cocoa
  powder

Preheat the oven to 350°F. Spray two 8-inch round cake pans with vegetable spray.

1. Make cake: In a large bowl and using a whisk or electric mixer, beat egg yolks, 2/3 cup sugar, and oil. With a wooden spoon, stir in yogurt, cocoa, cake meal, and potato starch until combined.
2. In another bowl, beat 4 egg whites until they are foamy. Gradually add 1/3 cup sugar, beating until stiff peaks form. Stir one quarter of the egg whites into the batter. Gently fold in the remaining egg whites just until blended. Divide the batter between the prepared cake pans.
3. Bake in the centre of the oven for 15 to 20 minutes or until a tester inserted in the centre comes out clean.
4. Let the pans cool on a wire rack.
5. Make icing: In the top of a double boiler over simmering water or in a bowl that sits on a pot of simmering water, combine 3 egg whites, 3/4 cup sugar, and water. With an electric mixer, beat for approximately 8 minutes or until the mixture is thickened and soft peaks form. Remove the pan from the heat; beat for 1 to 2 minutes or until stiff peaks form. Sift the cocoa into the icing; beat it in until it is thoroughly blended.
6. Place one cake layer on a cake platter. Spread some of the icing over top. Place the second cake layer on top of the first. Ice the top and sides.

marble mocha cheesecake

This delicious cheesecake was in my *Enlightened Home Cooking* and it remains one of my favourites. I created a brownie base that is delicious with the creamy cheese filling.

MAKES 12 SERVINGS

NUTRITIONAL ANALYSIS
PER SERVING
Energy 271 calories
Protein 7 g
Fat, total 11 g
Fat, saturated 4.4 g
Carbohydrates 36 g
Fibre 1 g
Cholesterol 54 mg

CRUST
3/4 cup granulated sugar
1/3 cup unsweetened cocoa
   powder
1/3 cup low-fat sour cream
1/4 cup vegetable oil
1 large egg
1 tsp vanilla
1/3 cup matzo cake meal
2 tbsp potato starch

FILLING
1 1/2 tsp instant coffee
   granules
2 tsp hot water
1 2/3 cups smooth 5% ricotta
   cheese
1/3 cup light cream cheese,
   softened
1/3 cup low-fat sour cream
1 large egg

1 tsp vanilla
3/4 cup granulated sugar
1 tbsp potato starch

SWIRL
3 tbsp semi-sweet chocolate
   chips
1 tbsp water

Preheat the oven to 350°F. Spray an 8-inch springform pan with vegetable spray.

1. Make crust: In a bowl and using a whisk or electric mixer, combine sugar, cocoa, sour cream, oil, egg, and vanilla. In another bowl, stir together the cake meal and potato starch; with a wooden spoon, stir the mixture into the cocoa mixture just until everything is mixed. Pour the mixture into a prepared pan. Bake in the centre of the oven for 15 minutes.

2. Make filling: Dissolve the instant coffee in hot water. Place it in a food processor along with ricotta cheese, cream cheese, sour cream, egg, vanilla, sugar, and potato starch; purée the mixture until it is smooth. Pour it into the pan.

3. Make swirl: In microwavable bowl, combine the chocolate chips and water. Microwave on medium-high for approximately 40 seconds or until the chips begin to melt. Stir the mixture until it is smooth. Drizzle it over the cheesecake batter. Using a butter knife, swirl the chocolate into the batter.

4. Bake in the centre of the oven for 35 to 40 minutes or until the cake is just slightly loose at the centre.

5. Run a butter knife around the edge of the cake. Let it cool on a wire rack until it is room temperature. Chill.

NUTRITION WATCH
Most cheesecakes served at Passover are high in fat because they're made of 35% MF cream cheese and lots of whole eggs. By substituting ricotta for the cream cheese and using only 1 egg, you reduce the calories, fat, and cholesterol.

TIP
You can use 2% cottage cheese instead of the ricotta, but be sure to process well to make the batter smooth.

apple and dried cranberry crisp

This Passover crisp tastes as delicious as the ones I make for the rest of the year. The topping is so crunchy and delicious.

MAKES 8 SERVINGS

NUTRITIONAL ANALYSIS
PER SERVING
Energy 243 calories
Protein 1.3 g
Fat, total 6.4 g
Fat, saturated 0.5 g
Carbohydrates 45 g
Fibre 2.0 g
Cholesterol 0 mg

NUTRITION WATCH
One piece of matzo is approximately 110 calories and 0.5 g
of fat. Avoid egg matzo,
which contains extra calories,
fat, and cholesterol from the
addition of the eggs.

TIP
Be sure to use matzo meal,
not matzo cake meal, for the
topping. It is not as fine and
makes a better texture.

CRISP
3 cups sliced and peeled apples
1/3 cup granulated sugar
1/3 cup dried cranberries
1/4 cup peach or apricot jam
3 tbsp matzo meal
1/2 tsp ground cinnamon
1 tbsp lemon juice

TOPPING
1/2 cup matzo meal
1/2 cup packed brown sugar
1/4 cup chopped pecans
1/2 tsp ground cinnamon
2 tbsp vegetable oil
2 tbsp water

Preheat the oven to 350°F. Spray an 8-inch square pan with vegetable spray.

1. In a bowl, stir together apples, sugar, cranberries, jam, matzo meal, cinnamon, and lemon juice. Pour the mixture into a prepared pan.
2. Make topping: In a bowl, stir together matzo meal, brown sugar, pecans, cinnamon, oil, and water until crumbly. Sprinkle the mixture over the fruit mixture.
3. Bake in the centre of the oven for 40 minutes or until the top is golden.
4. Serve warm.

chocolate cream cheese pie

This is a creamy chocolatey pie, with a firm crust thanks to the cake meal. Serve it with Vanilla Cream (see page 241).

CRUST

1 cup matzo cake meal

1/3 cup granulated sugar

2 tbsp unsweetened cocoa powder

3 tbsp water

3 tbsp vegetable oil

FILLING

1 1/2 cups smooth 5% ricotta cheese

2 1/2 oz light cream cheese, softened

3/4 cup granulated sugar

1/4 cup unsweetened cocoa powder

1 large egg

1 1/2 tbsp potato starch

1/3 cup low-fat sour cream

2 tbsp semi-sweet chocolate chips

Preheat the oven to 350°F. Spray a 9-inch pie plate with vegetable spray.

1. Make crust: In a bowl, stir together cake meal, sugar, cocoa, water, and oil until everything is well mixed. Pat the mixture into a prepared pie plate.
2. Make filling: In a food processor, combine ricotta cheese, cream cheese, sugar, cocoa, egg, potato starch, and sour cream; purée until the mixture is smooth. Pour it into the crust. Sprinkle with chocolate chips.
3. Bake in the centre of the oven for 30 to 35 minutes or until the filling is set.
4. Let the pan cool on a wire rack. Chill.

MAKES 12 SERVINGS

NUTRITIONAL ANALYSIS PER SERVING

Energy 220 calories

Protein 6.3 g

Fat, total 8.3 g

Fat, saturated 3.4 g

Carbohydrates 30 g

Fibre 1.2 g

Cholesterol 32 mg

NUTRITION WATCH

Ricotta cheese is a good source of calcium.

TIPS

Cottage cheese (2% MF) can replace ricotta cheese. Purée it well until the curds are smooth, and add another 2 tsp potato starch.

Sour cream can be replaced with low-fat yogurt.

cheesecake squares

These cheesecake squares are moist and delicious. The crust tastes just like graham crackers.

BASE

1 cup matzo cake meal

1/3 cup granulated sugar

1/4 cup water

1 tbsp vegetable oil

FILLING

3/4 cup smooth 5% ricotta
   cheese

3/4 cup low-fat cottage
   cheese

1/2 cup granulated sugar

1 1/2 tbsp potato starch

1 large egg

1 tsp vanilla

GLAZE

2 oz semi-sweet chocolate or
   1/4 cup chocolate chips

2 tbsp water

Preheat the oven to 350°F. Spray an 8-inch square baking dish with vegetable spray.

1. Make base: In a bowl, stir together cake meal, sugar, water, and oil until combined. Press the mixture onto the bottom of a prepared dish.
2. Make filling: In a food processor, combine ricotta cheese, cottage cheese, sugar, potato starch, egg, and vanilla; purée the mixture until it is smooth. Pour it into the dish.
3. Bake in the centre of the oven for 15 to 20 minutes or until the centre is slightly loose. Let it cool for 20 minutes before glazing.
4. Make glaze: In microwavable bowl, combine the chocolate and water. Heat it on medium-high for 40 seconds or until the chocolate begins to melt. Stir until it is melted. Spread it over the squares. Chill for 1 hour.

brownies with marshmallow and chocolate topping

I pack these brownies for my children's lunch during Passover week. All the other kids want the recipe!

3/4 cup granulated sugar
1/3 cup unsweetened cocoa powder
1/8 tsp salt
1/3 cup low-fat sour cream
1/4 cup vegetable oil
1 large egg
1 tsp vanilla
1/3 cup matzo cake meal
1 tbsp potato starch
1/3 cup miniature marshmallows
2 tbsp semi-sweet chocolate chips

Preheat the oven to 350°F. Spray an 8-inch square baking dish with vegetable spray.

1. In a bowl and using a whisk or electric mixer, combine sugar, cocoa, salt, sour cream, oil, egg, and vanilla.
2. In another bowl, stir together cake meal and potato starch. With a wooden spoon, stir the mixture into the cocoa mixture just until everything is combined. Pour the mixture into a prepared dish.
3. Bake in the centre of the oven for 10 minutes or just until the brownies are slightly loose at the centre.
4. Sprinkle with marshmallows and chocolate chips. Bake for another 5 minutes.
5. Let the pan cool on a wire rack.

MAKES 12 SERVINGS

NUTRITIONAL ANALYSIS PER SERVING
Energy 139 calories
Protein 1.6 g
Fat, total 6.3 g
Fat, saturated 1.3 g
Carbohydrates 19 g
Fibre 1 g
Cholesterol 20 mg

NUTRITION WATCH
I buy brownies from a Passover bakery and they are delicious but loaded with fat and calories due to the large amounts of oil and eggs used. My version is much healthier.

TIPS
Buy Passover marshmallows, because the regular kind contains corn syrup, which is not to be used.

If you only can find large marshmallows, use scissors to cut them into smaller pieces.

mocha brownies

NUTRITIONAL ANALYSIS
PER SERVING
Energy 160 calories
Protein 1.9 g
Fat, total 6.3 g
Fat, saturated 1.2 g
Carbohydrates 24 g
Fibre 1.0 g
Cholesterol 18 mg

NUTRITION WATCH
You can substitute butter or
margarine for the oil.
Remember, whichever you
choose, the amount of calories and fat is approximately
the same; butter, though, contains saturated fat.

TIP
If you don't have brewed
coffee on hand, dissolve 1 tsp
instant coffee in 1 tbsp boiling
water.

These are my adult version of brownies. They are moist and chocolatey and definitely hit the spot.

1/4 cup semi-sweet chocolate chips
1/4 cup water
1 tbsp strong brewed coffee
1 cup granulated sugar
1/4 cup unsweetened cocoa powder
1 large egg
1 large egg white
1/4 cup vegetable oil
2/3 cup matzo cake meal

Preheat the oven to 350°F. Spray an 8-inch square baking dish with vegetable spray.

1. Combine chocolate chips, water, and coffee in a microwavable bowl. On medium-high, microwave for 40 seconds or until the chips begin to melt. Stir the mixture until it is smooth.
2. In a large bowl and using a whisk or electric mixer, combine sugar, cocoa, egg, egg white, and oil. Add the chocolate mixture. With a wooden spoon, stir in the cake meal just until everything is combined.
3. Pour the mixture into a prepared baking dish.
4. Bake in the centre of the oven for 15 to 18 minutes or until the centre is still slightly loose.
5. Let the pan cool on a wire rack.

apricot orange sponge cake with orange glaze

Passover sponge cakes are traditionally made with a large amount of egg yolks, oil, and egg whites beaten and then folded into the batter. My version uses two yolks and most of the leavening power comes from the egg whites. Its combination of apricot and orange is wonderful. Serve with Mango Coulis (see page 243) or top with sliced strawberries.

CAKE
2 large egg yolks
1 tbsp finely grated orange
   rind
1/2 cup orange juice
1/3 cup vegetable oil
1/4 cup orange juice
   concentrate

3/4 cup granulated sugar
2/3 cup matzo cake meal
2/3 cup potato starch
6 large egg whites
1/2 cup granulated sugar
1/2 cup diced dried apricots

GLAZE
1 tbsp orange juice
   concentrate
1/4 cup Passover icing sugar

Preheat the oven to 350°F. Use a 9-inch springform pan, not sprayed.

1. Make cake: In a large bowl and using a whisk or electric mixer, combine yolks, orange rind, orange juice, oil, orange juice concentrate, and 3/4 cup sugar.
2. In another bowl, stir together the cake meal and potato starch. With a wooden spoon, stir the mixture into the orange mixture just until everything is combined.
3. In a separate bowl, beat the egg whites until they are foamy. Gradually add 1/2 cup sugar, beating until stiff peaks form. Stir the apricots and one quarter of the egg whites into the cake batter. Gently fold in the remaining egg whites just until blended. Pour the mixture into a pan.
4. Bake in the centre of the oven for 30 to 35 minutes or until a tester inserted in the centre comes out clean.
5. Let the pan cool on a wire rack. Remove the side of the pan.
6. Make glaze: Mix orange juice concentrate and icing sugar until the mixture is smooth. Pour it over the cake.

MAKES 12 SERVINGS

NUTRITIONAL ANALYSIS
PER SERVING
Energy 236 calories
Protein 3.3 g
Fat, total 7.0 g
Fat, saturated 0.7 g
Carbohydrates 40 g
Fibre 1 g
Cholesterol 35 mg

NUTRITION WATCH
I have greatly reduced the fat and cholesterol of this sponge cake by using fewer egg yolks and more egg whites. The flavour is enhanced by the orange and apricot.

TIP
During Passover, you cannot use cream of tartar because it is made during alcohol distillation and contains baking soda, which is a leavening agent. I find that the whites will still beat well without the cream of tartar, but if you're having trouble try adding 2 tsp of lemon juice.

banana roll with chocolate filling

This is a delicious and moist cake that you would never believe has so little fat and calories.

MAKES 8 SERVINGS

NUTRITIONAL ANALYSIS
PER SERVING
Energy 200 calories
Protein 3.4 g
Fat, total 2.9 g
Fat, saturated 1.5 g
Carbohydrates 40 g
Fibre 1.2 g
Cholesterol 27 mg

NUTRITION WATCH
Bananas are high in carbohydrates, low in fat, and rich
in potassium and vitamin C.

TIP
Garnish with Passover icing
sugar and sliced bananas that
have been rubbed with lemon
juice to prevent browning.

CAKE
1 ripe medium (1/3 cup) banana,
   mashed
1/2 cup granulated sugar
1 large egg
1 1/2 tsp vanilla
1/4 cup matzo cake meal
2 tbsp potato starch
4 large egg whites

1/2 cup granulated sugar
2 tbsp Passover icing sugar

FILLING
1/4 cup semi-sweet chocolate chips
2 tbsp water
1 ripe small banana
Passover icing sugar

Preheat the oven to 350°F. Line a 10-inch × 15-inch jelly roll pan with parchment paper and spray with vegetable spray.

1. In a large bowl and using a whisk or electric mixer, beat mashed banana, 1/2 cup sugar, egg, and vanilla.
2. In another bowl, stir together cake meal and potato starch.
3. In a separate bowl, beat the egg whites until they are foamy. Gradually add 1/2 cup sugar, beating until stiff peaks form.
4. With a wooden spoon, stir the cake meal mixture into the banana mixture. Stir one quarter of the egg whites into the cake batter. Gently fold in the remaining egg whites just until combined. Pour the mixture into a prepared pan, spreading it evenly.
5. Bake in the centre of the oven for 12 to 15 minutes or until a tester comes out dry. Let the pan cool on a wire rack.
6. Dust the cake with 2 tbsp icing sugar and invert it onto a clean tea towel. Remove the pan and peel off the parchment paper.
7. Make filling: Melt the chocolate chips with water in microwave for approximately 40 seconds. Stir to melt it, and spread it over the surface. Thinly slice the banana; scatter the slices over the cake. Starting from the short end, gently roll up the cake, with the help of the tea towel. Transfer it to a serving platter, seam side down. Garnish with icing sugar.

chocolate jelly roll

This is a simple jelly roll cake lined with a creamy ricotta cheese filling and sprinkled with chocolate chips.

CAKE

1/2 cup granulated sugar

1/4 cup unsweetened cocoa powder

1/4 cup water

1 large egg

1/4 cup matzo cake meal

2 tbsp potato starch

3 large egg whites

1/3 cup granulated sugar

Passover icing sugar

FILLING

1 1/4 cups smooth 5% ricotta cheese

2/3 cup Passover icing sugar

1 tsp vanilla

3 tbsp semi-sweet chocolate chips

Preheat the oven to 350°F. Line a 15-inch × 10-inch jelly roll pan with parchment paper and spray it with vegetable spray.

1. Make cake: In a bowl and using a whisk or electric mixer, combine 1/2 cup sugar, cocoa, water, and egg.
2. In another bowl, stir together the cake meal and potato starch. With a wooden spoon, stir the mixture into the cocoa mixture just until everything is combined.
3. In another bowl, beat the egg whites until they are foamy. Gradually add 1/3 cup sugar, beating until stiff peaks form. Stir one quarter of the egg whites into the batter. Gently fold in the remaining egg whites just until combined. Pour the mixture into a prepared pan, spreading it evenly.
4. Bake in the centre of the oven for 12 to 15 minutes or until a tester comes out dry.
5. Let the pan cool on a wire rack.
6. Make filling: In a food processor, combine ricotta cheese, icing sugar, and vanilla; purée the mixture until it is smooth. Stir in the chocolate chips.
7. Dust the cake with 2 tbsp icing sugar. Invert it onto a clean tea towel. Remove pan and peel off the parchment paper. Spread the filling over the surface. Starting from the short end, gently roll up the cake, with the help of the tea towel. Transfer the cake to a serving platter, seam side down. Sprinkle it with icing sugar.

NUTRITIONAL ANALYSIS PER SERVING

Energy 258 calories

Protein 7.6 g

Fat, total 5.3 g

Fat, saturated 3 g

Carbohydrates 45 g

Fibre 1.3 g

Cholesterol 38 mg

NUTRITION WATCH

Ricotta cheese is a wonderful substitute for cream cheese in baking. It contains only 5% MF and is creamy and smooth.

TIP

Regular icing sugar cannot be used during Passover because it contains corn-starch to prevent the sugar from getting lumpy. But there is an icing sugar that contains potato starch, which works well.

coffee pecan mandel brot

MAKES ABOUT
30 COOKIES

NUTRITIONAL ANALYSIS
PER SERVING
Energy 88 calories
Protein 1 g
Fat, total 3.4 g
Fat, saturated 0.3 g
Carbohydrates 13 g
Fibre 0.3 g
Cholesterol 7 mg

NUTRITION WATCH
Egg white binds the cookie
batter and lowers the fat and
cholesterol in this recipe.

TIP
If you don't have instant
coffee, use 2 tbsp strong
brewed coffee.

When I was testing Passover desserts, I found my favourite were the mandel brot. I actually prefer them to regular cookies!

1 1/2 tbsp instant coffee granules
2 tbsp hot water
3/4 cup packed brown sugar
1/2 cup granulated sugar
1/4 cup vegetable oil
1 large egg
1 large egg white
1 1/2 cups matzo cake meal
1/2 cup potato starch
1/2 cup toasted chopped pecans

Preheat the oven to 350°F. Spray a large cookie sheet with vegetable spray.

1. Dissolve the instant coffee in hot water.
2. In a large bowl and using a whisk or electric mixer, combine coffee, brown sugar, sugar, oil, egg, and egg white.
3. In another bowl, stir together cake meal, potato starch, and pecans. Stir the mixture into the coffee mixture just until combined. Divide it in half. Form two logs, each approximately 3 inches wide and 8 inches long. Transfer the logs to the cookie sheet.
4. Bake in the centre of the oven for 20 minutes. Remove the sheet from the oven and let the logs cool on the sheet for 5 minutes.
5. Transfer the logs to a cutting board. Slice them on the diagonal into 1/2-inch thick cookies.
6. Place the cookies flat on the sheet. Bake for 15 minutes longer.

chocolate chip mandel brot

These cookies are wonderful after a heavy Passover meal. My children love them during the day with a glass of milk.

3/4 cup granulated sugar
1/4 cup vegetable oil
2 large eggs
2 tsp vanilla
1 1/2 cups matzo cake meal
1/3 cup potato starch
1/3 cup semi-sweet chocolate chips

Preheat the oven to 350°F. Spray a large cookie sheet with vegetable spray.

1. In a large bowl and using a whisk or electric mixer, combine sugar, oil, eggs, and vanilla.
2. In another bowl, stir together cake meal, potato starch, and chocolate chips. Stir the mixture into the sugar mixture until combined. Divide it in half. Form two logs, each approximately 3 inches wide and 8 inches long. Transfer the logs to the cookie sheet.
3. Bake in the centre of the oven for 15 minutes. Remove the sheet from the oven and let the logs cool on the sheet for 5 minutes.
4. Transfer the logs to a cutting board. Slice them on the diagonal into 1/2-inch thick cookies.
5. Place the cookies flat on the sheet. Bake for 15 minutes longer.

MAKES ABOUT
30 COOKIES

NUTRITIONAL ANALYSIS
PER SERVING
Energy 75 calories
Protein 2.4 g
Fat, total 2.7 g
Fat, saturated 0.6 g
Carbohydrates 11.7 g
Fibre 0.2 g
Cholesterol 14 mg

NUTRITION WATCH
Feel free to substitute 1 egg
with 2 egg whites in order to
lower the fat and cholesterol
in your baking.

TIP
If you can find other flavours
of Passover chocolate chips,
such as mint, orange, or
white, try them, too.

orange cranberry mandel brot

The combination of orange and dried cranberries is delicious in this light cookie.

MAKES ABOUT
30 COOKIES

NUTRITIONAL ANALYSIS
PER SERVING
Energy 73 calories
Protein 1 g
Fat, total 1.9 g
Fat, saturated 0.4 g
Carbohydrates 13 g
Fibre 0.4 g
Cholesterol 14 mg

NUTRITION WATCH
Dried fruit is a concentrated
form of energy. Eat it in moderation because the calories
are more dense.

TIP
Use orange juice concentrate
for the most intense orange
flavour. Keep a can in the
freezer to use only for baking
or cooking.

3/4 cup granulated sugar
1/4 cup margarine or butter
1/4 cup orange juice concentrate
2 large eggs
1 tbsp finely grated orange rind
2 tsp vanilla
1 1/2 cups matzo cake meal
1/2 cup potato starch
1/2 cup dried cranberries

Preheat the oven to 350°F. Spray a large cookie sheet with vegetable spray.

1. In a large bowl and using a whisk or electric mixer, combine sugar, margarine, orange juice con-centrate, eggs, orange rind, and vanilla.
2. In another bowl, stir together cake meal, potato starch, and cranberries. Stir the mixture into the sugar mixture until combined. Divide it in half. Form two logs, each approximately 3 inches wide and 8 inches long. Transfer the logs to the cookie sheet.
3. Bake in the centre of the oven for 15 minutes. Remove the sheet from the oven and let the logs cool on the sheet for 5 minutes.
4. Transfer the logs to a cutting board. Slice them on the diagonal into 1/2-inch thick cookies.
5. Place the cookies flat on the sheet. Bake for 15 minutes longer.

other divine desserts

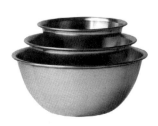

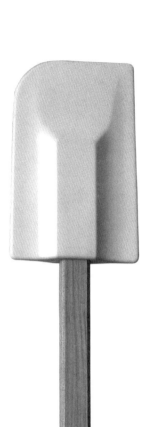

tips for divine light phyllo pastries

1. Phyllo pastry is found in the freezer section of the grocery store. It consists of many layers of paper-thin pastry that's perfect for baking. Thaw it at room temperature or overnight in the refrigerator.

2. The key with phyllo is to work quickly. After removing the number of sheets you need, cover the remaining phyllo with plastic wrap and a slightly wet towel. If it dries out, it can no longer be used.

3. Keep the fat to a minimum when baking with phyllo by coating every other sheet with vegetable spray. Always spray the outer sheet so it browns well while it is being baked.

4. Phyllo desserts can be prepared in advance, sprayed with vegetable spray, covered tightly with plastic wrap, and frozen until ready to bake. Just add 5 to 10 minutes extra baking time.

5. Bake phyllo desserts on a cookie sheet lined with parchment paper that has been sprayed with vegetable spray.

6. Phyllo is ready when the crust becomes golden and crisp. Cut slices with a sharp or serrated knife.

7. For jelly rolls, it is best to use a 15-inch × 10-inch jelly roll pan. Line the pan with parchment paper and spray it with vegetable spray to avoid any sticking.

8. Mix the wet ingredients first and then mix the dry ingredients so they are ready to be added. Beat egg whites until they are foamy, adding the sugar gradually until stiff peaks form. Then add the flour mixture to the wet ingredients and mix just until the flour is incorporated. Fold in the whites just until they are blended. Do not overfold or the egg whites will deflate. Spread the batter immediately evenly in the pan and bake it in the centre of the oven for even baking.

9. Many of the fillings in these recipes are based on ricotta cheese. Be sure to process the filling well to make the batter as smooth as possible. The fillings will roll more easily if they have been chilled.

10. To test doneness, place a toothpick or tester into cake. The cake is ready if the tester comes out dry and clean.

11. Cool the cake on a wire rack until it is room temperature. Sprinkle 2 tbsp icing sugar over top and then invert it onto a clean tea towel. The icing sugar prevents the cake from sticking. Peel away the parchment paper, spread the filling onto the cake, and begin to roll, using the tea towel to assist. Roll gently until the whole cake is rolled; then carefully place it on a serving dish, seam side down. Chill.

12. If the cake cracks while rolling, it may not have been baked long enough and is still slightly wet, or it may have been baked too long and is too dry. Prevent cracks by checking the cake regularly with a tester a few minutes before the baking time is up. Cover any cracks with sprinkled icing sugar or cocoa.

13. Serve jelly rolls at room temperature or chilled.

lemon tiramisu

In *Enlightened Home Cooking,* I created a Chocolate Coffee Tiramisu that was luscious.
You never knew it didn't contain mascarpone cheese. I adapted it to a Lemon Tiramisu that
I think may even be better.

1 3/4 cups smooth 5% ricotta cheese

4 oz light cream cheese, softened

1/2 cup granulated sugar

1 tbsp finely grated lemon rind

1/3 cup fresh lemon juice

1 large egg yolk

3 large egg whites

1/4 tsp cream of tartar

1/3 cup granulated sugar

1/2 cup boiling water

3 tbsp fresh lemon juice

3 tbsp granulated sugar

20 3-inch ladyfinger cookies

Spray a 9-inch square cake pan or decorative serving dish with vegetable spray.

1. In a food processor, combine ricotta cheese, cream cheese, 1/2 cup sugar, lemon rind, lemon
   juice, and yolk; purée the mixture until it is smooth. Transfer it to a large bowl.
2. In another bowl, beat the egg whites with the cream of tartar until they are foamy. Gradually add
   1/3 cup sugar, beating until stiff peaks form. Stir one quarter of the egg whites into the ricotta
   mixture. Gently fold in the remaining egg whites just until blended.
3. In a bowl, whisk together water, lemon juice, and 3 tbsp sugar. Dip each ladyfinger in the mixture
   just enough to moisten it and place it in the bottom of the baking dish. Pour half the ricotta-
   lemon mixture over the ladyfingers. Repeat layers. Chill at least 2 hours.

MAKES 12 SERVINGS

NUTRITIONAL ANALYSIS
PER SERVING
Energy 204 calories
Protein 7.8 g
Fat, total 6.3 g
Fat, saturated 3.4 g
Carbohydrates 29 g
Fibre 0.2 g
Cholesterol 88 mg

NUTRITION WATCH
Thanks to ricotta cheese and
light cream cheese, there is
little fat in this wonderful traditional dessert. Mascarpone
cheese has 14 g of fat per
2 tbsp; ricotta has only 3 g
of fat per 2 tbsp.

TIPS
Process the cheeses well
until the batter is no longer
grainy.

Be sure to beat the egg
whites and sugar well until
all the granules are dissolved.

Use only fresh lemon juice.

baked alaska

For this traditional dessert, frozen yogurt or sorbet replaces the ice cream, reducing the fat.

MAKES 12 SERVINGS

NUTRITIONAL ANALYSIS
PER SERVING
Energy 228 calories
Protein 6.4 g
Fat, total 1.6 g
Fat, saturated 0.9 g
Carbohydrates 47 g
Fibre 0.7 g
Cholesterol 21 mg

NUTRITION WATCH
One half cup of frozen yogurt
has approximately 3 g of fat
depending on the flavour;
1/2 cup of ice cream can have
between 14 to 20 g of fat.
What a difference!

TIPS
To make this dish even more
dramatic, use different
flavours of yogurt or sorbet.
Try 1 cup of four different
flavours, totalling 4 cups.

You can refreeze any left-
overs, but this cake tastes
best right out of the oven.

You can always buy store-
bought sponge cake if you
don't have time to make your
own.

CAKE
1 large egg
1/3 cup granulated sugar
1/3 cup low-fat milk
1 1/2 tsp vanilla
2/3 cup all-purpose flour
1/2 tsp baking powder

1/8 tsp salt
3 large egg whites
1/4 tsp cream of tartar
1/4 cup granulated sugar
2 tbsp icing sugar
4 cups frozen yogurt or
   sorbet, any flavour, softened

TOPPING
3 large egg whites
1 cup granulated sugar
1/4 cup water
1/4 tsp cream of tartar

Preheat oven to 350°F. Line 15-inch × 10-inch jelly roll pan with parchment paper and spray with vegetable spray.

1. Make cake: In a bowl, whisk together egg, 1/3 cup sugar, milk, and vanilla. In another bowl, stir together flour, baking powder, and salt; with a wooden spoon, stir the mixture in the egg mixture.
2. In a separate bowl, beat the egg whites with the cream of tartar until foamy. Gradually add 1/4 cup sugar, beating until stiff peaks form. Stir one quarter of the egg whites into the batter. Gently stir in remaining egg whites. Pour onto a prepared pan, spreading it evenly.
3. Bake in centre of oven for 12 to 15 minutes or until tester comes out dry. Let cool on a rack.
4. Dust cake with icing sugar. Invert onto clean tea towel. Remove pan and peel off parchment paper. Cut cake in thirds lengthwise, then in thirds crosswise to create nine squares. Cut each square on the diagonal to create two triangles.
5. Line a 6-cup bowl with plastic wrap, with a 6-inch overhang all around. Line it with some triangles placed end to end, trimming as necessary to cover the inside of bowl completely. Pack frozen yogurt into bowl. Place additional triangles on top to encase yogurt completely. Trim any bits that extend beyond the covering. Fold wrap over the dessert. Freeze for at least 2 hours.
6. Preheat the oven to 450°F.
7. Make topping: In the top of a double boiler, mix egg whites, sugar, water, and cream of tartar. Beat with electric beater for approximately 7 minutes, until soft peaks form. Remove pan from heat and beat for 2 more minutes until mixture is stiff.
8. Remove bowl from freezer and remove plastic wrap. Invert cake onto pan and remove bowl. Using a spatula, spread topping over surface of cake. Bake in the centre of the oven for 3–5 minutes or until cake is golden. Serve immediately.

raspberry charlotte

A charlotte is a classic moulded dessert lined with sponge cake or ladyfingers and filled with a mixture of fruit, custard, and whipping cream. My version uses low-fat condensed milk and egg whites to get a delicious flavour and texture.

CRUST

3 tbsp raspberry jam

2 tbsp hot water

about 40 3″ ladyfinger cookies

FILLING

1 can (1 1/4 cups) low-fat
   sweetened condensed milk

2 cups smooth 5% ricotta cheese

2 cups fresh or frozen raspberries

1/3 cup granulated sugar

1 tbsp unflavoured gelatin powder

3 tbsp cold water

3 large egg whites

1/4 tsp cream of tartar

1/4 cup granulated sugar

Use an ungreased 8-inch springform pan.

1. Make crust: In a small bowl, stir together jam and water. Brush the ladyfingers with the mixture. Line the bottom of the pan with some of the ladyfingers. Break them to fit as necessary.

2. Make filling: In a food processor, combine condensed milk, ricotta cheese, raspberries, and 1/3 cup sugar; purée the mixture until it is smooth. In a small microwavable bowl, combine gelatin and water; let sit for 2 minutes. Microwave on high for 20 seconds. Stir it until it is smooth. With the motor running, add the gelatin to food processor though feed tube. Transfer the mixture to a large bowl.

3. In another bowl, beat the egg whites with the cream of tartar until they are foamy. Gradually add 1/4 cup sugar, beating until stiff peaks form. Stir one quarter of the egg whites into the ricotta-gelatin mixture. Gently fold in the remaining egg whites just until combined. Pour the mixture into the pan. Place the remaining ladyfingers against the wall of the pan with the flat part of the cookie facing out, pushing through the mousse filling.

4. Chill for at least 3 hours.

NUTRITIONAL ANALYSIS
PER SERVING

Energy 279 calories

Protein 10 g

Fat, total 5.7 g

Fat, saturated 3.2 g

Carbohydrates 47 g

Fibre 1.5 g

Cholesterol 61 mg

NUTRITION WATCH

Two tablespoons of regular condensed milk has 3 g of fat. The low-fat version has only 1.5 g of fat.

TIPS

If you're using frozen berries, measure them while they're frozen, then thaw and drain them well.

Condensed milk is a mixture of cow's milk and sugar. It's heated until about 60% of the water evaporates, which results in a sticky, sweet mixture, delicious for baking. The low-fat version is just as good, if not better.

date turnovers

MAKES 16 SERVINGS

NUTRITIONAL ANALYSIS
PER SERVING

Energy 91 calories

Protein 1.4 g

Fat, total 3.3 g

Fat, saturated 0.8 g

Carbohydrates 14 g

Fibre 0.6 g

Cholesterol 2.5 mg

NUTRITION WATCH

Dates are a good source of protein and iron. I enjoy them as a mid-day snack for a quick energy and complex carbohydrate boost.

TIPS

I like to keep my dates in the freezer. I buy them at a bulk food store and use them as needed.

Use scissors to cut dried fruit.

Turnovers are traditionally made with a lot of butter and flour. This dough uses some light cream cheese with a small amount of oil and butter. The texture is still light and much lower in fat and calories.

PASTRY

2 1/2 oz light cream cheese, softened

1/4 cup granulated sugar

2 tbsp vegetable oil

1 tbsp margarine or butter

1 cup all-purpose flour

1 to 2 tbsp water

FILLING

3 oz (2/3 cup) chopped pitted dates

1/2 cup orange juice

1 tsp finely grated orange rind

Preheat the oven to 375°F. Spray a cookie sheet with vegetable spray.

1. Make pastry: In a food processor, combine cream cheese, sugar, oil, and margarine; purée the mixture until it is smooth. Add the flour and 1 tbsp water. Pulse until the mixture is crumbly, adding more water as necessary. Form the dough into a ball and wrap in plastic wrap. Chill for 20 minutes.

2. Make filling: In a saucepan, combine dates, orange juice, and orange rind. Bring to a boil over medium-high heat; reduce heat and simmer for 5 to 8 minutes or until the liquid is absorbed. Mash the mixture until it is smooth. Let it cool while you prepare the dough.

3. Between two sheets of floured waxed paper, roll the dough to 1/8 inch thick. Using a 2-inch round cutter, cut out 16 circles. Re-roll scraps.

4. Place 1 1/2 tsp date purée on each pastry circle, off centre. Fold in half. Press the edges, using a little water to seal. Place them on the prepared cookie sheet. Repeat with the remaining filling and pastry.

5. Bake in the centre of the oven for 15 to 20 minutes or until the turnovers are golden.

tropical phyllo strudel

Traditionally strudel is a type of pastry made of many layers of very thin dough spread with a filling. It's rarely made at home because of the time and complexity it requires. Phyllo pastry from the refrigerator section of the supermarket is a wonderful substitute. The fresh tropical fruits in this strudel make it extra special. Serve with Mango Coulis (see page 243).

2 cups (approximately 1 large)
   diced fresh mango
2 cups diced fresh pineapple
1/3 cup dried cranberries
1/3 cup granulated sugar
1/4 cup toasted coconut
1 tbsp all-purpose flour
1/2 tsp ground cinnamon
6 sheets phyllo pastry
Vegetable spray

Preheat the oven to 375°F. Spray a large cookie sheet with vegetable spray.

1. In a bowl, stir together mango, pineapple, cranberries, sugar, coconut, flour, and cinnamon.
2. On a work surface, layer one sheet of phyllo on top of the other. Spray the surface with vegetable spray. Top with two more sheets of phyllo. Spray. Top with the last two sheets of phyllo. Spread the filling over the surface, leaving a 1-inch border on all sides. Starting at the short end, roll the phyllo several times away from you. Fold the left and right edges of phyllo in and over the filling. Continue to roll the strudel. Transfer it to the cookie sheet, seam side down. Spray the entire strudel.
3. Bake in the centre of the oven for 25 to 30 minutes or until it is golden and crisp.

NUTRITIONAL ANALYSIS PER SERVING

Energy 164 calories

Protein 1.7 g

Fat, total 2.8 g

Fat, saturated 1.7 g

Carbohydrates 33 g

Fibre 2.4 g

Cholesterol 0

NUTRITION WATCH

The fresh fruits in this strudel supply an abundance of vitamins and other nutrients, as well as containing very little to no fat. Mangoes and pineapple contain vitamins A and C.

TIPS

Keep the phyllo in the freezer and leave it at room temperature or overnight in the refrigerator until it is thawed before using.

Work quickly with phyllo and keep the sheets not being used covered with a tea towel.

Rewrap unused phyllo and refreeze it.

phyllo strudel with cherries

MAKES 8 SERVINGS

NUTRITIONAL ANALYSIS
PER SERVING
Energy 191 calories
Protein 6 g
Fat, total 5.7 g
Fat, saturated 3.1 g
Carbohydrates 29 g
Fibre 0.6 g
Cholesterol 42 mg

NUTRITION WATCH
Cherries contain small
amounts of vitamins and are
a good source of potassium.

TIP
Pitted cherries are not always
easy to find. I usually use the
ones that come unsweetened
in a jar, not packed in heavy
syrup.

The combination of a cream-cheese filling and sour pitted cherries is delicious in this phyllo strudel. Serve it with frozen yogurt or Raspberry Coulis (see page 242).

4 oz light cream cheese, softened
3/4 cup smooth 5% ricotta cheese
2/3 cup granulated sugar
2 tsp all-purpose flour
1 tsp vanilla
1 large egg
5 sheets phyllo pastry
Vegetable spray
2/3 cup drained canned pitted cherries

Preheat the oven to 375°F. Spray a large cookie sheet with vegetable spray.

1. In a food processor, combine cream cheese, ricotta cheese, sugar, flour, vanilla, and egg; purée the mixture until it is smooth.
2. Layer two sheets of phyllo one on top of the other. Spray with vegetable spray. Layer another two on top; spray. Place the final sheet on top. Spread the cheese mixture over the surface, leaving a 1-inch border on all sides. Scatter the cherries over top. Starting at the short end, roll the phyllo several times away from you. Fold the left and right edges of the phyllo in and over the filling. Continue to roll the strudel. Transfer it to a cookie sheet, seam side down. Spray the entire strudel with vegetable spray.
3. Bake in the centre of the oven for 25 to 30 minutes or until the strudel is golden and crisp.

baklava pecan phyllo squares

Baklava, popular in Greece and Turkey, is a sweet dessert that usually consists of many layers of butter-drenched phyllo pastry, spices, and nuts, with a lemon-honey syrup poured over top. My recipe uses no fat except for vegetable spray. The filling is what makes this dessert so divine.

HONEY MIXTURE
1/3 cup granulated sugar
1/4 cup water
3 tbsp honey
1 1/2 tbsp lemon juice

FILLING
1/2 cup Grape-Nuts cereal
1/2 cup raisins
1/2 cup chopped toasted pecans
1/3 cup packed brown sugar
1/2 tsp ground cinnamon
4 sheets phyllo pastry
Vegetable spray

Preheat the oven to 350°F.
Spray an 8-inch square baking dish with vegetable spray.

1. In a saucepan, combine sugar, water, honey, and lemon juice; cook the mixture over medium heat for 5 minutes.
2. In a bowl, stir together cereal, raisins, pecans, brown sugar, cinnamon, and 3 tbsp of the honey mixture.
3. On a work surface, cut each phyllo sheet into quarters. Layer two squares in a prepared dish one on top of the other. Spray with vegetable spray. Repeat the process until eight squares have been layered. Scatter the nut mixture over top. Layer the remaining phyllo squares on top, spraying after every other sheet. Spray the top.
4. Bake for 20 to 25 minutes or until the phyllo is golden. Reheat remaining honey mixture if necessary and pour it over the hot baklava. Let them cool on a wire rack.

MAKES 12 SERVINGS

NUTRITIONAL ANALYSIS
PER SERVING
Energy 155 calories
Protein 1.6 g
Fat, total 4.1 g
Fat, saturated 0.4 g
Carbohydrates 28 g
Fibre 1.3 g
Cholesterol 0

NUTRITION WATCH
If traditional baklava is drenched with butter, you can just imagine the calories and fat. One tablespoon of butter contains 100 calories and 11 g of fat.

TIP
Grape-Nuts cereal is a wonderful wheat and toasted barley cereal with virtually no fat. I like it because it gives a dessert the texture of chopped nuts, without the excess calories or fat.

phyllo apple cheese pie

MAKES 12 SERVINGS

NUTRITIONAL ANALYSIS
PER SERVING
Energy 138 calories
Protein 3.3 g
Fat, total 3.2 g
Fat, saturated 1.6 g
Carbohydrates 24 g
Fibre 1 g
Cholesterol 25 mg

NUTRITION WATCH
Apples are a good source of
vitamins A and C. Have one
during the day to supply some
fibre and carbohydrates.

TIP
Use a sweet, tasty, firm apple
such as Mutsu, Royal Gala, or
Spy. Avoid those that are too
soft, such as McIntosh or
Golden Delicious.

This version of a phyllo apple pie with a cream-cheese filling makes a regular apple pie seem ordinary. I like to serve it warm, with sorbet or with Vanilla Cream (see page 241).

CHEESE MIXTURE	APPLE MIXTURE
3 oz light cream cheese, softened	4 cups diced peeled apples
1/2 cup smooth 5% ricotta cheese	1/3 cup packed brown sugar
1/3 cup granulated sugar	1 tbsp all-purpose flour
1 large egg	1/2 tsp ground cinnamon
2 tsp all-purpose flour	6 sheets phyllo pastry
1 tsp vanilla	Vegetable spray

Preheat the oven to 350°F. Spray a 9-inch springform pan with vegetable spray.

1. In a food processor, combine cream cheese, ricotta cheese, sugar, egg, flour, and vanilla; purée the mixture until it is smooth.
2. In a bowl, stir together apples, brown sugar, flour, and cinnamon.
3. Place two sheets of the phyllo in a prepared pan, letting the excess hang over sides. Spray with vegetable spray. Place two more sheets in the pan, arranging them so the excess falls over different sides of the pan from first two sheets. Spray. Place the last two sheets of the phyllo in the pan. Place the apple mixture in the pan. Pour the cheese mixture over top. Fold the excess phyllo up and over top of the filling so it is completely enclosed. Spray with vegetable spray.
4. Bake for 35 to 40 minutes or until the phyllo is golden. Let it cool on a wire rack.

banana chocolate roll

This jelly roll looks dramatic with its spiral design — white sponge roll, fudge filling, dotted with bananas!

CAKE

3/4 cup (about 2 medium) mashed ripe
   banana
1/2 cup granulated sugar
1 large egg
1 tsp vanilla
3/4 cup all-purpose flour
1/2 tsp baking soda
3 large egg whites
1/4 tsp cream of tartar
1/4 cup granulated sugar

FILLING

1/2 cup smooth 5% ricotta cheese
2 oz light cream cheese, softened
1/3 cup granulated sugar
2 tbsp unsweetened cocoa powder
2 tbsp low-fat sour cream
2 tbsp icing sugar
1 small banana

Preheat the oven to 350°F. Line a 15-inch × 10-inch jelly roll pan with parchment paper and spray it with vegetable spray.

1. Make cake: In large bowl and using a whisk or electric mixer, beat mashed banana, 1/2 cup sugar, egg, and vanilla.

2. In another bowl, stir together flour and baking soda.

3. In a separate bowl, beat the egg whites with the cream of tartar until they are foamy. Gradually add 1/4 cup sugar, beating until stiff peaks form.

4. With a wooden spoon, stir the flour mixture into the banana mixture just until combined. Stir one quarter of the egg whites into the cake batter. Gently fold in the remaining egg whites just until blended. Pour the batter onto a prepared pan, spreading it evenly.

5. Place the pan in the centre of the oven for 12 to 15 minutes or until a tester comes out dry. Let the pan cool on a wire rack.

6. Make filling: In a food processor, combine ricotta cheese, cream cheese, sugar, cocoa, and sour cream; purée the mixture until it is smooth.

7. Dust cake with icing sugar. Invert onto a tea towel. Remove pan and peel off parchment paper. Spread filling over surface. Thinly slice the banana; scatter over cake. Starting from the short end, gently roll up the cake with the help of the tea towel. Transfer it to a serving platter, seam side down.

NUTRITIONAL ANALYSIS
PER SERVING
Energy 257 calories
Protein 6.6 g
Fat, total 3.8 g
Fat, saturated 2.1 g
Carbohydrates 49 g
Fibre 1.6 g
Cholesterol 37 mg

NUTRITION WATCH
Bananas are high in carbohydrates, low in protein and
fat, and rich in potassium
and vitamin C.

TIPS
For the best-tasting bananas
for cooking, store overripe
ones in the freezer. When you
need them, just defrost them
and use.

To ripen bananas, place them
in a perforated brown paper
bag for a few days.

apple cinnamon cream roll

Taking a basic jelly roll recipe and adding different flavours and textures can create a wide variety of incredible desserts, like this one.

MAKES 8 SERVINGS

NUTRITIONAL ANALYSIS
PER SERVING
Energy 245 calories
Protein 6.6 g
Fat, total 4.3 g
Fat, saturated 2.2 g
Carbohydrates 45 g
Fibre 0.8 g
Cholesterol 38 mg

NUTRITION WATCH
Jelly rolls are low in fat and
calories because there is no
fat added to the batter. But be
careful of the traditional
ones, which are filled with
whipping cream or butter
icings.

TIP
Use a firm, sweet-tasting
apple for maximum flavour.
Mutsu, Spy, and Royal Gala
are good choices.

CAKE
1/2 cup packed brown sugar
1/3 cup unsweetened
   applesauce
1 large egg
1/2 tsp ground cinnamon
2/3 cup all-purpose flour
1/2 tsp baking powder

3 large egg whites
1/4 tsp cream of tartar
1/4 cup granulated sugar

FILLING
1 tsp margarine or butter
1 cup diced peeled apple
1 tbsp packed brown sugar

1/4 tsp ground cinnamon
3/4 cup smooth 5% ricotta
   cheese
2 oz light cream cheese,
   softened
1/3 cup granulated sugar
2 tbsp icing sugar

Preheat the oven to 350°F. Line a 15-inch × 10-inch jelly roll pan with parchment paper and spray with vegetable spray.

1. Make cake: In a large bowl and using a whisk or electric mixer, beat brown sugar, applesauce, egg, and cinnamon.
2. In another bowl, stir together flour and baking powder; with a wooden spoon, stir the mixture into the applesauce mixture just until it is combined.
3. In another bowl, beat the egg whites with cream of tartar until they are foamy. Gradually add 1/4 cup sugar, beating until stiff peaks form. Stir one quarter of the egg whites into the apple-sauce mixture. Gently fold in the remaining whites just until blended. Pour the mixture onto a prepared pan, spreading it evenly.
4. Place the pan in the centre of the oven and bake for 12 minutes or until a tester inserted in the centre comes out clean. Let the pan cool on a wire rack.
5. Make filling: In a frying pan, melt the margarine over medium-high heat; cook the apples, brown sugar, and cinnamon for 3 minutes. Let it cool while you prepare the filling.
6. In a food processor, combine ricotta cheese, cream cheese, and sugar; purée the mixture until it is smooth. Stir in the apple mixture.
7. Dust the cake with icing sugar, and invert it onto a clean tea towel. Remove the pan and peel off the parchment paper. Spread the filling over the surface. Starting from the short end, gently roll up the cake with the help of the tea towel. Transfer it to a serving platter, seam side down.

chocolate chip marble roll

This is a marbled jelly roll, filled with a creamy cheese filling and dotted with chocolate chips.

MAKES 8 SERVINGS

CAKE

2 large egg yolks

2/3 cup granulated sugar

1/3 cup low-fat milk

1 tsp vanilla

1/3 cup all-purpose flour

1/4 tsp baking powder

1/4 cup all-purpose flour

3 tbsp unsweetened
   cocoa powder

1/4 tsp baking powder

3 large egg whites

1/4 tsp cream of tartar

1/4 cup granulated sugar

FILLING

1 cup smooth 5% ricotta
   cheese

1 oz light cream cheese,
   softened

1/3 cup granulated sugar

1 tsp vanilla

2 tbsp semi-sweet chocolate
   chips

2 tbsp icing sugar

Preheat the oven to 350°F. Line a 15-inch × 10-inch jelly roll pan with parchment paper and spray with vegetable spray.

1. Make cake: In a bowl and using a whisk or electric mixer, beat egg yolks, 2/3 cup sugar, milk, and vanilla. Pour half the mixture into another bowl. In one bowl, with a wooden spoon stir in 1/3 cup flour and 1/4 tsp baking powder. In the other bowl, with a wooden spoon stir in 1/4 cup flour, cocoa, and 1/4 tsp baking powder just until mixed.

2. In a third bowl, beat the egg whites with the cream of tartar until they are foamy. Gradually add 1/4 cup sugar, beating until stiff peaks form. Fold half the egg whites into the white batter and half into the brown batter just until blended.

3. Drop batters in mounds onto a prepared pan, alternating colours. Spread it evenly, swirling the two batters gently.

4. Place the pan in the centre of the oven and bake for 12 to 14 minutes or until a tester inserted in the centre comes out clean. Let the pan cool on a wire rack.

5. Make filling: In a food processor, combine ricotta cheese, cream cheese, sugar, and vanilla; purée the mixture until it is smooth. Stir in chocolate chips.

6. Dust cake with icing sugar. Invert onto a tea towel. Remove pan and peel off parchment paper. Spread filling over surface. Starting from the short end, gently roll up the cake with the help of the tea towel. Transfer it to a serving platter, seam side down. Chill for 1 hour.

NUTRITIONAL ANALYSIS
PER SERVING

Energy 265 calories

Protein 7.7 g

Fat, total 5.6 g

Fat, saturated 3 g

Carbohydrates 46 g

Fibre 1.1 g

Cholesterol 65 mg

NUTRITION WATCH

One egg contains 75 calories, 6 g of protein, 5 g of fat, and 180 mg of cholesterol. Eggs are a healthy part of a diet, if not consumed in excess.

TIP

When folding egg whites into the batter, mix only until the whites are blended in. If you overfold, they'll lose their volume and the texture of the cake won't be as light.

orange roll with mandarin cheese filling

NUTRITIONAL ANALYSIS
PER SERVING
Energy 203 calories
Protein 4.6 g
Fat, total 2.7 g
Fat, saturated 1.4 g
Carbohydrates 40 g
Fibre 0.7 g
Cholesterol 33 mg

NUTRITION WATCH
Mandarin oranges are an
excellent source of vitamin C
and contain some vitamin A.

TIP
You can use fresh mandarins,
tangerines, or clementines
when they are in season —
peel them and remove all the
seeds. Be sure they are
sweet!

This is a light and refreshing dessert, especially after a heavy meal. With every mouthful, you get a piece of sweet mandarin orange.

CAKE
1/3 cup granulated sugar
2 tsp finely grated orange rind
1/4 cup orange juice
1 large egg
2/3 cup all-purpose flour
1/2 tsp baking powder

3 large egg whites
1/4 tsp cream of tartar
1/4 cup granulated sugar

FILLING
3 oz light cream cheese, softened
2/3 cup icing sugar

2 tbsp orange juice concentrate
1 tsp finely grated orange rind
1/2 cup drained canned mandarin oranges
2 tbsp icing sugar

Preheat the oven to 350°F. Line a 15-inch × 10-inch jelly roll pan with parchment paper and spray with vegetable spray.

1. Make cake: In a large bowl, whisk together 1/3 cup sugar, orange rind and juice, and egg. With a wooden spoon, stir in the flour, and baking powder just until mixed.
2. In another bowl, beat the egg whites with the cream of tartar until they are foamy. Gradually add 1/4 cup sugar, beating until stiff peaks form. Stir one quarter of the egg whites into the orange mixture. Gently fold in the remaining whites just until blended. Pour the mixture onto a prepared pan, spreading it evenly.
3. Place the pan in the centre of the oven and bake for 10 to 12 minutes or until a tester inserted in the centre comes out clean. Let the pan cool on a wire rack.
4. Make filling: In a food processor, combine cream cheese, icing sugar, orange juice concentrate, and orange rind; purée the mixture until it is smooth. Stir in mandarin oranges.
5. Dust the cake with icing sugar and invert it onto a clean tea towel. Remove the pan and peel off the parchment paper. Spread the filling over the surface. Starting from the short end, gently roll up the cake with the help of the tea towel. Transfer it to a serving platter, seam side down.

gingerbread roll

Gingerbread flavouring is associated with a gingery taste accompanied by molasses, coffee, or honey. Its distinct flavour makes for a unique jelly roll dessert.

CAKE

2 tsp instant coffee
   granules

3 tbsp hot water

2/3 cup packed brown sugar

1 tbsp molasses

1 tsp vanilla

1 large egg

3/4 cup all-purpose flour

1/2 tsp ground cinnamon

1/4 tsp ground ginger

1/8 tsp allspice

3 large egg whites

1/4 tsp cream of tartar

1/4 cup granulated sugar

FILLING

1 cup smooth 5% ricotta
   cheese

2 oz light cream cheese,
   softened

1/2 cup packed brown sugar

2 tbsp molasses

2 tbsp icing sugar

Preheat the oven to 350°F. Line a 15-inch × 10-inch jelly roll pan with parchment paper and spray with vegetable spray.

1. Dissolve the coffee in hot water.
2. In a large bowl, whisk together coffee, brown sugar, molasses, vanilla, and egg. In another bowl, stir together flour, cinnamon, ginger, and allspice; with a wooden spoon, stir this mixture into the molasses mixture until mixed.
3. In another bowl, beat the egg whites with the cream of tartar until they are foamy. Gradually add the sugar, beating until stiff peaks form. Stir one quarter of the egg whites into the cake batter. Gently fold in the remaining egg whites just until blended. Pour the mixture onto a prepared pan, spreading it evenly.
4. Place the pan in the centre of the oven and bake for 10 to 12 minutes or until a tester inserted in the centre comes out clean. Let the pan cool on a wire rack.
5. Make filling: In a food processor, combine ricotta cheese, cream cheese, brown sugar, and molasses; purée the mixture until it is smooth.
6. Dust the cake with icing sugar and invert it onto a clean tea towel. Remove the pan and peel off the parchment paper. Spread the filling over the surface. Starting from the short end, gently roll up the cake with the help of the tea towel. Transfer it to a serving platter, seam side down.

MAKES 8 SERVINGS

NUTRITIONAL ANALYSIS
PER SERVING
Energy 294 calories
Protein 7.6 g
Fat, total 4.4 g
Fat, saturated 2.5 g
Carbohydrates 56 g
Fibre 0.4 g
Cholesterol 40 mg

NUTRITION WATCH
Molasses contains iron, calcium, and phosphorous.

TIP
There are three different kinds of molasses: extra light, dark, and blackstrap. Light comes from the first boiling, dark from the second, and blackstrap from the third. Dark is traditionally used in desserts.

lemon roll with lemon curd filling

This double-hit of a lemon dessert makes lemon lovers like me think we're in heaven.

MAKES 8 SERVINGS

NUTRITIONAL ANALYSIS
PER SERVING
Energy 260 calories
Protein 3.8 g
Fat, total 1.4 g
Fat, saturated 0.6 g
Carbohydrates 58 g
Fibre 0.5 g
Cholesterol 29 mg

NUTRITION WATCH
If you're looking for a cake
with the lowest fat, calories,
and cholesterol, your best
selection is a jelly roll cake.
It's one of the few cakes without any added fat. Beware of
the fillings in commercial
ones, though, because they
usually contain whipping
cream and buttered icings.

TIP
Use only freshly squeezed
lemon juice when the recipe
depends on the lemon for its
primary flavour. Bottled lemon
juice is fine when a small
amount is called for.

FILLING
3/4 cup granulated sugar
3 tbsp cornstarch
1/3 cup fresh lemon juice
1/3 cup water
1 oz light cream cheese,
    softened

CAKE
2/3 cup granulated sugar
2 tsp finely grated lemon
    rind
1/4 cup fresh lemon juice
1 large egg
3/4 cup all-purpose flour
1/2 tsp baking powder

3 large egg whites
1/4 tsp cream of tartar
1/4 cup granulated sugar
2 tbsp icing sugar

GLAZE
3 tbsp icing sugar
1 tbsp fresh lemon juice

Preheat the oven to 350°F. Line a 15-inch × 10-inch jelly roll pan with parchment paper and spray with vegetable spray.

1. Make filling: In a small saucepan off the heat, whisk together sugar, cornstarch, lemon juice, and water until smooth. Cook the mixture over medium heat, whisking constantly, for 2 to 3 minutes or until it has thickened. Remove the pan from the heat; whisk in the cream cheese until it has dissolved. Transfer the mixture to a bowl. Cover the surface with a piece of plastic wrap. Let it chill while you prepare the cake.

2. Make cake: In a large bowl, whisk together sugar, lemon rind, lemon juice, and egg. With a wooden spoon, stir in the flour, and baking powder until mixed.

3. In another bowl, beat the egg whites with the cream of tartar until they are foamy. Gradually add 1/4 cup sugar, beating until stiff peaks form. Stir one quarter of the egg whites into the cake batter. Gently fold in the remaining egg whites just until blended. Pour the mixture onto a prepared pan, spreading it evenly.

4. Place the pan in the centre of the oven and bake for 10 minutes or until a tester inserted in the centre comes out clean. Let the pan cool on a wire rack.

5. Dust the cake with icing sugar and invert it onto a clean tea towel. Remove the pan and peel off the parchment paper. Spread the filling over the surface. Starting from the short end, gently roll up the cake with the help of the tea towel. Transfer it to a serving platter, seam side down.

6. Make glaze: Whisk icing sugar and lemon juice together until smooth. Drizzle over lemon roll.

muffins, scones, and loaf cakes

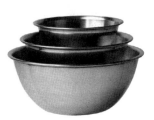

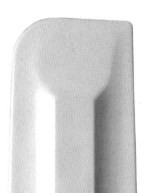

tips for divine light muffins, scones, and loaf cakes

1. Read the recipe before starting, making certain all of the ingredients are available or that you have ingredients that can substitute.

2. For the best results, the butter, margarine, and eggs should be at room temperature. It's not necessary, though.

3. Preheat the oven and set the rack in the middle for even baking.

4. Always coat the muffin tins and loaf pans with either vegetable spray, which is easiest, or butter or margarine. This prevents sticking. You can also use paper liners.

5. Follow the recipe carefully, step by step. Always mix the wet ingredients thoroughly, then add the dry ingredients. The key is not to overmix the entire batter or your muffins or loaf cakes will be dry and tough. Use a whisk, hand beater, or food processor. Mix just until the flour is no longer lumpy and seems to be blended with the liquid ingredients.

6. If you're using a food processor to mix the ingredients, be careful not to overprocess the dry ingredients. I use an on-off pulsing to incorporate the dry ingredients just until the flour is no longer visible.

7. Some of the recipes make larger muffins than others. Just divide the batter among the 12 muffin cups accordingly, using standard muffin baking tins.

8. I use a 9-inch x 5-inch loaf pan for all my loaf cakes.

9. Watch the baking of low-fat muffins and loaf cakes very carefully since they have no excess fat that would tolerate excess baking. At least 5 minutes before the baking time is finished, insert a toothpick or cake tester to check for doneness. The tester should come out clean and dry. If it is still slightly wet, bake for just another 2 to 3 minutes and watch carefully. The muffins and cakes should be golden brown, firm to the touch, and come away from the sides of the pan.

10. Muffins taste the best when they're still warm. I freeze them for later in a freezer plastic bag for up to 3 months. Warm them in a toaster oven at 350°F for 5 minutes.

11. Loaf cakes can also be frozen, well wrapped, for up to 3 months.

12. I often interchange muffin and loaf cake recipes, but must watch the baking times carefully. Muffins take approximately between 18 and 25 minutes, whereas loaf cakes can take between 35 to 55 minutes. I always use the tester to check for doneness.

13. Don't store muffins or loaf cakes in the refrigerator because they become stale and dry faster. Leave them on the counter or in the freezer.

banana bran apricot muffins

This variation on the standard bran muffin is outstanding. I pack these for my children's lunches.

1 medium (1/3 cup) ripe banana, mashed
3/4 cup granulated sugar
1 cup low-fat milk
1/4 cup vegetable oil
1 large egg
1 tsp vanilla
1 cup all-purpose flour
3/4 cup natural bran
3/4 cup chopped dried apricots
1 tsp baking powder
1 tsp baking soda

Preheat the oven to 350°F. Spray a 12-cup muffin pan with vegetable spray.

1. In a large bowl and using a whisk or electric beaters, combine banana, sugar, milk, oil, egg, and vanilla.
2. In another bowl, stir together flour, bran, apricots, baking powder, and baking soda. With a wooden spoon, stir the mixture into the banana mixture just until everything is combined. Divide the mixture among the prepared muffin cups.
3. Bake for 15 to 18 minutes or until a tester inserted into the middle of a muffin comes out dry.

NUTRITIONAL ANALYSIS
PER SERVING
Energy 187 calories
Protein 3.4 g
Fat, total 5.5 g
Fat, saturated 0.6 g
Carbohydrates 31 g
Fibre 2.8 g
Cholesterol 19 mg

NUTRITION WATCH
Bran is a good source of carbohydrates, calcium, phosphorous, and fibre. The best nutritional source is from natural bran, but bran buds and flakes are also a good source.

TIP
Freeze leftover bananas to use for baking. Just defrost and mash.

cappuccino chip muffins

NUTRITIONAL ANALYSIS
PER SERVING
Energy 171 calories
Protein 2.6 g
Fat, total 6.3 g
Fat, saturated 1.2 g
Carbohydrates 26 g
Fibre 0.6 g
Cholesterol 18 mg

NUTRITION WATCH
I'm always asked what are
the best oils to use. Use
those with the least amount
of saturated fats and the
highest amount of mono-
unsaturated fats: canola,
olive, or peanut oil.

TIP
If you don't have instant coffee on hand, just use 2 tbsp
left-over brewed.

The slight addition of coffee to your muffins perks them up. I love this as a late-morning snack.

1 tbsp instant coffee granules
2 tbsp hot water
2/3 cup low-fat milk
1/4 cup vegetable oil
1 large egg
1 1/2 tsp vanilla
3/4 cup granulated sugar
1 1/3 cups all-purpose flour
1/4 cup semi-sweet chocolate chips
1 1/2 tsp baking powder

Preheat the oven to 350°F. Spray a 12-cup muffin pan with vegetable spray.

1. Dissolve the instant coffee in hot water. In a large bowl and using a whisk or electric beaters, combine dissolved coffee, milk, oil, egg, vanilla, and sugar.
2. In another bowl, stir together flour, chocolate chips, and baking powder. With a wooden spoon, stir the mixture into the coffee mixture just until everything is combined. Divide the mixture among the prepared muffin cups.
3. Bake for 15 to 18 minutes or until a tester inserted into the middle of a muffin comes out dry.

banana peanut butter jam muffins

Forget the peanut butter and jam sandwiches. Try these great muffins. My kids devour them!

1 large (1/2 cup) ripe banana, mashed
3 tbsp smooth peanut butter
1 large egg
1/2 cup low-fat milk
2 tbsp vegetable oil
1 tsp vanilla
3/4 cup granulated sugar
1 1/4 cups all-purpose flour
1/2 cup bran flakes cereal or corn flakes cereal
1 1/2 tsp baking powder
1/2 tsp baking soda
3 tbsp raspberry jam

Preheat the oven to 350°F. Spray a 12-cup muffin pan with vegetable spray.

1. In a large bowl and using a whisk or electric beaters, combine banana, peanut butter, egg, milk, oil, vanilla, and sugar.
2. In another bowl, stir together flour, cereal, baking powder, and baking soda. With a wooden spoon, stir the mixture into the banana mixture just until everything is combined. Divide the mixture among the prepared muffin cups. Dollop a small amount of jam on top of each muffin.
3. Bake for 15 to 18 minutes or until a tester inserted into the middle of a muffin comes out dry.

MAKES 12 MUFFINS

NUTRITIONAL ANALYSIS PER SERVING

Energy 187 calories
Protein 3.5 g
Fat, total 5 g
Fat, saturated 0.7 g
Carbohydrates 32 g
Fibre 1.2 g
Cholesterol 18 mg

NUTRITION WATCH
Peanut butter, when combined with a bread or grain becomes a full protein — great for children who don't consume enough protein or who are vegetarians.

TIP
I use only pure smooth peanut butter that consists only of peanuts. Most commercial peanut butters have icing sugar added.

chocolate cheesecake muffins

MAKES 12 MUFFINS

NUTRITIONAL ANALYSIS
PER SERVING
Energy 201 calories
Protein 4.2 g
Fat, total 7.1 g
Fat, saturated 1.7 g
Carbohydrates 30 g
Fibre 1 g
Cholesterol 24 mg

NUTRITION WATCH
Light cream cheese is 25%
lower in fat than regular
cream cheese. Use it carefully.

TIPS
I usually make a double batch
of these muffins and freeze
them for school lunches and
dessert.

You can substitute low-fat
cottage cheese for the ricotta
cheese, but purée it well.

My children think I'm making Twinkies. These are divine treasures for young and old, with a creamy filling in every mouthful.

1 cup granulated sugar
1/3 cup unsweetened cocoa powder
1 cup low-fat yogurt
1/4 cup vegetable oil
1 tsp vanilla
1 large egg
3/4 cup all-purpose flour
1 1/2 tsp baking powder
2 oz light cream cheese, softened
1/3 cup smooth 5% ricotta cheese
1/3 cup icing sugar

Preheat the oven to 350°F. Spray a 12-cup muffin pan with vegetable spray.

1. In a large bowl and using a whisk or electric beaters, combine sugar, cocoa, yogurt, oil, vanilla, and egg.
2. In another bowl, stir together flour and baking powder. With a wooden spoon, stir the mixture into the cocoa mixture just until everything is combined. Divide half of the batter among the prepared muffin cups.
3. With clean beaters or in a food processor, beat cream cheese, ricotta cheese, and icing sugar until the mixture is smooth. Divide the cheese mixture among the muffin cups. Top with the remaining batter.
4. Bake for 20 to 25 minutes or until a tester inserted into the middle of a muffin comes out dry.

gingerbread date muffins

I've always enjoyed gingerbread cookies, so I took the flavouring and applied it to muffins. These may be even better than the cookies!

3/4 cup granulated sugar

2/3 cup low-fat yogurt

3 tbsp vegetable oil

3 tbsp molasses

1 large egg yolk

1 cup all-purpose flour

1 1/2 tsp baking powder

3/4 tsp ground cinnamon

1/4 tsp ground ginger

1/8 tsp allspice

1/2 cup chopped pitted dates

2 large egg whites

1/4 tsp cream of tartar

2 tbsp granulated sugar

Preheat the oven to 350°F. Spray a 12-cup muffin pan with vegetable spray.

1. In a large bowl and using a whisk or electric beaters, combine 3/4 cup sugar, yogurt, oil, molasses, and egg yolk.

2. In another bowl, stir together flour, baking powder, cinnamon, ginger, and allspice. With a wooden spoon, stir the mixture into the molasses mixture along with the dates, just until everything is combined.

3. In a clean bowl and using clean beaters, beat the egg whites with the cream of tartar until they are foamy. Gradually add 2 tbsp sugar, continuing to beat until stiff peaks form. Fold the mixture into the batter just until combined. Divide it among the prepared muffin cups.

4. Bake for 15 minutes or until a tester inserted into the middle of a muffin comes out dry.

MAKES 12 MUFFINS

NUTRITIONAL ANALYSIS
PER SERVING

Energy 156 calories

Protein 2.6 g

Fat, total 4.2 g

Fat, saturated 0.5 g

Carbohydrates 27 g

Fibre 0.4 g

Cholesterol 19 mg

NUTRITION WATCH

Molasses is rich in iron, calcium, and phosphorous.

TIPS

Don't worry if you're missing allspice. Try nutmeg or increase the amount of cinnamon.

The most common molasses is dark molasses, which is what is used in most traditional North American cooking.

apple butter streusel muffins

Apple butter is a thick, dark-brown preserve made by slowly cooking apples, sugar, spices, and cider, which is then puréed and strained. It has a more intense flavour than applesauce.

MAKES 12 MUFFINS

NUTRITIONAL ANALYSIS
PER SERVING
Energy 181 calories
Protein 2.3 g
Fat, total 3.5 g
Fat, saturated 0.4 g
Carbohydrates 35 g
Fibre 0.8 g
Cholesterol 18 mg

NUTRITION WATCH
Apple butter is a great substitute for a topping over toast
or breads, instead of butter or
cream cheese. It has no fat or
cholesterol.

TIPS
If you don't have apple butter,
use unsweetened applesauce.

Use a firm sweet apple for
the best flavour. I avoid
McIntosh and Gold Delicious
for cooking, and prefer Royal
Gala, Spy, and Mutsu.

TOPPING
3 tbsp packed brown sugar
3 tbsp Grape-Nuts cereal
2 tbsp all-purpose flour
1/4 tsp ground cinnamon
1 1/2 tsp vegetable oil
1 1/2 tsp water

MUFFINS
2/3 cup granulated sugar
1/4 cup packed brown sugar
1/2 cup low-fat milk
1/3 cup apple butter
2 tbsp vegetable oil
1 large egg
1 cup all-purpose flour
1 tsp baking powder
1/2 tsp baking soda
1/2 tsp ground cinnamon
3/4 cup chopped peeled apples
2 tsp all-purpose flour

Preheat the oven to 350°F. Spray a 12-cup muffin pan with vegetable spray.

1. Make topping: In a bowl, stir together brown sugar, cereal, flour, cinnamon, oil, and water just until crumbly. Set the mixture aside.
2. Make muffins: In a large bowl and using a whisk or electric beaters, combine sugar, brown sugar, milk, apple butter, oil, and egg.
3. In another bowl, stir together 1 cup flour, baking powder, baking soda, and cinnamon. With a wooden spoon, stir the mixture into the apple butter mixture just until everything is combined.
4. In a small bowl, stir together apples and 2 tsp flour; stir the mixture into the batter. Divide the batter among the prepared muffin cups. Sprinkle the topping evenly over top.
5. Bake for 18 to 20 minutes or until a tester inserted into the middle of a muffin comes out dry.

cranberry streusel muffins

Who says cranberries are only for the festive season? I keep a bag of frozen ones on hand. You don't need to thaw them.

TOPPING
2 tbsp quick-cooking oats
2 tbsp all-purpose flour
2 tbsp packed brown sugar
1/4 tsp ground cinnamon
2 tsp vegetable oil
1 tsp water

MUFFINS
3/4 cup granulated sugar
1/2 cup low-fat milk
1/4 cup vegetable oil
1 large egg
1 tsp vanilla
1 cup coarsely chopped
   cranberries
1 1/3 cups all-purpose flour
2 tsp baking powder

Preheat the oven to 350°F. Spray a 12-cup muffin pan with vegetable spray.

1. Make topping: In a small bowl, stir together oats, flour, brown sugar, cinnamon, oil, and water until the mixture is crumbly. Set it aside.
2. Make muffins: In a large bowl and using a whisk or electric beaters, combine sugar, milk, oil, egg, and vanilla. With a wooden spoon, stir in the cranberries.
3. In another bowl, stir together flour and baking powder. With a wooden spoon, stir the mixture into the cranberry mixture just until everything is combined. Divide the mixture among the prepared muffin cups. Sprinkle the topping evenly over top.
4. Bake for 18 to 20 minutes or until a tester inserted into the middle of a muffin comes out dry.

MAKES 12 MUFFINS

NUTRITIONAL ANALYSIS
PER SERVING
Energy 181 calories
Protein 2.6 g
Fat, total 6.1 g
Fat, saturated 0.6 g
Carbohydrates 29 g
Fibre 0.9 g
Cholesterol 18 mg

NUTRITION WATCH
Cranberries are very high in vitamin C. Dried cranberries are a concentrated form of nutrients, carbohydrates, and energy.

TIP
Because cranberries are so tart, I balance the flavour with a sweet cinnamon topping.

cranberry applesauce loaf

Cranberries and applesauce make a great combination. The addition of cinnamon gives the cake a real punch.

LOAF
3/4 cup granulated sugar
1 tsp ground cinnamon
1/2 cup unsweetened applesauce
1/4 cup vegetable oil
1 large egg
2 tsp vanilla
1/2 cup low-fat yogurt
1 1/3 cups all-purpose flour
1 1/2 tsp baking powder
1/2 tsp baking soda
1 cup fresh or frozen cranberries

TOPPING
1/4 cup quick-cooking oats
3 tbsp packed brown sugar
2 tbsp all-purpose flour
1/4 tsp ground cinnamon
2 tsp vegetable oil
1 tsp water

Preheat the oven to 350°F. Spray a 9-inch × 5-inch loaf pan with vegetable spray.

1. Make loaf: In a large bowl and using a whisk or electric mixer, combine sugar, cinnamon, applesauce, oil, egg, vanilla, and yogurt.
2. In another bowl, stir together flour, baking powder, baking soda, and cranberries. With a wooden spoon, stir the mixture into the applesauce mixture just until everything is combined. Pour the mixture into a prepared loaf pan.
3. Make topping: In a small bowl, stir together oats, brown sugar, flour, cinnamon, oil, and water until crumbly. Sprinkle the mixture over the batter.
4. Bake in the centre of the oven for 45 to 50 minutes or until a tester inserted in the middle comes out dry.
5. Let the pan cool on a wire rack.

fig banana loaf

Figs are a divine fruit with a soft flesh and many tiny edible seeds. I came up with this dessert when I tasted a similar recipe in a local coffee shop. But that one was filled with fat and calories!

6 oz (1 1/4 cup) dried figs, chopped
3/4 cup water
3/4 cup granulated sugar
1 large (1/2 cup mashed) ripe banana
1/4 cup vegetable oil
1 large egg
1 large egg white
2 tsp vanilla
1/2 cup low-fat yogurt
1 2/3 cups all-purpose flour
1 1/2 tsp baking powder
1 1/2 tsp ground cinnamon
1/2 tsp baking soda

Preheat the oven to 350°F. Spray a 9-inch × 5-inch loaf pan with vegetable spray.

1. In a small saucepan, combine figs and water. Bring to a boil; reduce heat to medium-low and simmer, uncovered, for 10 minutes, stirring occasionally. Remove the pan from the heat. Cool.
2. In a food processor, combine the fig mixture, sugar, banana, oil, egg, egg white, and vanilla; purée the mixture until it is smooth. Add yogurt, flour, baking powder, cinnamon, and baking soda; pulse on and off just until everything is combined. Pour the mixture into a prepared pan.
3. Bake in the centre of the oven for 50 minutes or until a tester inserted in the middle comes out dry.
4. Let the pan cool on a wire rack.

MAKES 16 HALF SLICES

NUTRITIONAL ANALYSIS
PER SERVING
Energy 164 calories
Protein 2.8 g
Fat, total 4.1 g
Fat, saturated 0.5 g
Carbohydrates 29 g
Fibre 1.9 g
Cholesterol 14 mg

NUTRITION WATCH
Figs are a good source of iron, calcium, and phosphorous. Great as a mid-day snack or dessert.

TIPS
Dry figs can be bought either in bulk or in a package. I often buy them in bulk and freeze them.

Fresh figs are sensational and available from June to September.

blueberry sour cream scones

A scone is a Scottish quick bread that shares its name with the place where Scottish kings were once crowned. The original recipes were made from oats and baked on a griddle. Today's are flour-based and baked in the oven. These ones have blueberries, which makes them wonderful.

1/2 cup granulated sugar
3 tbsp cold butter
1 large egg
1 tsp vanilla
1 cup all-purpose flour
1 1/2 tsp baking powder
1/3 cup low-fat sour cream
1/2 cup fresh or frozen blueberries

Preheat the oven to 400°F. Spray a baking sheet with vegetable spray.

1. In a food processor, combine sugar, butter, egg, and vanilla; pulse on and off just until the mixture is crumbly. Add flour, baking powder, and sour cream; pulse on and off just until everything is combined. Stir in the blueberries.
2. Drop the batter on the baking sheet in 10 equal amounts.
3. Bake in the centre of the oven for 12 to 15 minutes or until the scones are golden. Serve them warm or at room temperature.

NUTRITIONAL ANALYSIS
PER SERVING
Energy 139 calories
Protein 2.3 g
Fat, total 4.6 g
Fat, saturated 2.7 g
Carbohydrates 22 g
Fibre 0.4 g
Cholesterol 33 mg

NUTRITION WATCH
Scones are traditionally made with a fair amount of butter and often served with extra butter or Devon cream, which make them unbelievably high in calories and fat. This recipe uses low-fat sour cream and only a little fat. I sometimes serve them with a small amount of jam.

TIPS
These scones are best with fresh berries. But if you're using frozen berries, measure them while they're still frozen, then defrost and drain them well.

You can use raspberries as well.

apricot orange scones

The combination of orange and dried apricots makes for a distinctive breakfast snack. The citrus flavour is highlighted by the addition of orange rind and orange juice concentrate.

1/2 cup granulated sugar
3 tbsp cold butter
1 large egg
1/3 cup evaporated skim milk
2 tbsp orange juice concentrate
2 tsp finely grated orange rind
1 tsp vanilla
1 cup all-purpose flour
1/3 cup diced dried apricots
1 1/2 tsp baking powder
1/8 tsp salt

Preheat the oven to 400°F. Spray a baking sheet with vegetable spray.

1. In a food processor, combine sugar, butter, egg, evaporated milk, orange juice concentrate, orange rind, and vanilla; pulse on and off just until everything is mixed. Add flour, baking powder, and salt; pulse on and off just until they are combined. Stir in apricots.
2. Drop the batter on the baking sheet in 10 equal amounts.
3. Bake in the centre of the oven for 10 to 12 minutes or until the scones are golden. Serve them warm or at room temperature.

MAKES 10 SCONES

NUTRITIONAL ANALYSIS
PER SERVING
Energy 153 g
Protein 2.9 g
Fat, total 4.1 g
Fat, saturated 2.3 g
Carbohydrates 26 g
Fibre 0.7 g
Cholesterol 31 mg

NUTRITION WATCH
Evaporated milk is canned unsweetened milk that has 60% of the water removed. Vitamin D is added for extra nutritional value. The skim milk version has almost no fat, whereas the whole milk version has almost 8% fat.

TIP
Evaporated milk gives the scones a creamy texture without using heavy cream or more butter. If you can't find skim you can use 2% evaporated milk.

the cookie jar

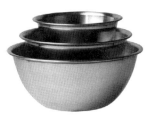

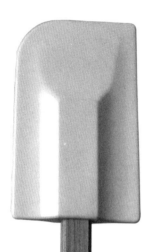

tips for divine light cookies

1. The basic cookie types used in this section are biscotti; drop cookies, which are dropped by the spoonful onto a baking sheet; rolled, chilled dough cookies; pressed cookies; and meringue cookies.

2. Preheat the oven. It's best if the ingredients are at room temperature.

3. You can substitute oil, butter, and margarine for one another. Oil gives a cookie a crispier texture and butter a softer texture. Use a whisk, hand beater, or food processor to mix cookies.

4. Mix the wet ingredients first, then add the dry ingredients and mix just until flour is incorporated. Do not overmix or the cookies will be tough.

5. Use nonstick baking sheets sprayed with vegetable spray, or line the sheet with parchment paper before spraying. Meringue cookies should always be placed on parchment paper to avoid sticking (but no spray is necessary).

6. I like to put the baking sheet in the centre of the oven rather than at the bottom because cookies usually burn at the bottom. The heat is more even in the centre of the oven.

7. The cookies are done when they have a golden bottom and the edges are brown. For a crisper cookie, bake a few minutes longer than the required time; for a softer chewier cookie, bake to the minimum time specified. Place the baking sheet on a rack to cool for a few minutes, then with a spatula place the cookies directly on the rack and let them cool until they are room temperature before storing.

8. Cookies are best eaten the day they are baked. But if you want to store them, most will keep fresh for a few days at room temperature in an airtight container or box, and for a few weeks in the freezer. To freeze, wrap them in plastic wrap and then in foil, and place them in freezer bags. They're great if reheated in a 400°F oven for approximately 5 minutes. Do not store cookies in the refrigerator.

9. Cookie dough, except for meringues, can be frozen and then baked frozen. Add a couple of minutes to the baking time.

10. Biscotti are twice-baked Italian cookies. They are formed into logs and placed on a greased baking sheet. They are usually baked for approximately 20 minutes, brought out on a rack to cool for 5 minutes, then sliced into 1/2-inch slices, turned onto their sides, and baked again for 15 to 20 minutes. The longer they bake the crisper they become.

11. The longer that meringues stay in the oven, the drier and chewier they become. You can leave them in the oven with the heat off, even as long as overnight.

apricot jam cranberry rugelach

I get weak at the knees when I think about rugelach. They are crisp, buttery, and melt in your mouth. But I usually avoid them because traditional recipes are loaded with fat. Not these. These ones are creamy, yet light.

2 oz light cream cheese
1/2 cup granulated sugar
1/4 cup vegetable oil
1 1/2 cups all-purpose flour
1/4 cup low-fat yogurt
1/3 cup apricot or raspberry jam
1/3 cup packed brown sugar
1/3 cup dried cranberries
1/2 tsp ground cinnamon

Preheat the oven to 350°F. Spray a baking sheet with vegetable spray.

1. In a food processor, purée cream cheese, sugar, and oil until smooth. Add flour and yogurt; pulse on and off until the mixture is crumbly. Remove the dough from the food processor. Form it into two balls and wrap them in plastic wrap. Chill at least 20 minutes.
2. Between two sheets of floured waxed paper, roll one ball into a circle 1/8-inch thick. Spread half the jam over top and sprinkle with half the brown sugar, cranberries, and cinnamon.
   With a sharp knife, cut the circle into 10 wedges. From the wide, outside edge, roll each wedge toward the centre; shape it into a crescent, and place it on a prepared baking sheet.
3. Repeat with the remaining dough, jam, brown sugar, cranberries, and cinnamon.
4. Bake for 20 minutes or until the rugelach are golden brown.

MAKES 20 COOKIES

NUTRITIONAL ANALYSIS
PER COOKIE
Energy 121 calories
Protein 1.5 g
Fat, total 3.4 g
Fat, saturated 0.6 g
Carbohydrates 21 g
Fibre 0.5 g
Cholesterol 1.8 mg

NUTRITION WATCH
Dried cranberries are loaded with vitamin C and are a wonderful source of energy.

TIP
If the jam is hard to spread, microwaving it for 30 seconds will soften it.

chocolate chocolate rugelach

MAKES ABOUT
22 COOKIES

NUTRITIONAL ANALYSIS
PER COOKIE
Energy 103 calories
Protein 1.4 g
Fat, total 3.3 g
Fat, saturated 0.9 g
Carbohydrates 17 g
Fibre 0.6 g
Cholesterol 1.3 mg

NUTRITION WATCH
I always tell people not to
deprive themselves of
dessert. Just try to practise
moderation. At least with
these cookies, there is no
room for guilt.

TIP
If you prefer the wedge
shape, follow the procedure
in Apricot Jam Cranberry
Rugelach (page 219).

A Hanukkah tradition, these cookies can include a variety of fillings with a rich cream cheese dough. If you adore rugelach, wait until you try the double-hit of chocolate in these. Try not to eat the whole batch in one sitting!

1 1/2 oz light cream cheese
1/2 cup granulated sugar
2 tbsp vegetable oil
2 tbsp margarine or butter
1 1/4 cups all-purpose flour
3 tbsp unsweetened cocoa powder
1/4 cup low-fat yogurt
1/2 cup packed brown sugar
3 tbsp semi-sweet chocolate chips
1 tbsp unsweetened cocoa powder
1/2 tsp ground cinnamon

Preheat the oven to 350°F. Spray baking sheet with vegetable spray.

1. In a food processor, purée cream cheese, sugar, oil, and margarine until the mixture is smooth. Add flour, 3 tbsp cocoa, and yogurt; pulse on and off until the dough is crumbly. Remove it from the food processor. Form the dough into two balls and wrap them with plastic wrap. Chill at least 20 minutes.
2. In a small bowl, stir together brown sugar, chocolate chips, 1 tbsp cocoa, and cinnamon.
3. Between two sheets of floured waxed paper, roll one ball into an approximately 12-inch × 8-inch rectangle, 1/4-inch thick. Sprinkle it with filling. From the long end, roll it up tightly. With a sharp knife, cut the log into 1/2-inch thick slices. Place them on the prepared baking sheet.
4. Repeat with remaining dough and filling.
5. Bake for 15 to 18 minutes or until the rugelach are golden brown on the bottom.

holiday cut-out cookies

These are cookies that kids love to have a hand in preparing. Use cut-outs for the holiday season. For different colours, add a drop or two of food colouring and let the kids decorate them with sprinkles, sugar, cinnamon, chocolate chips, jam, and anything else they want.

2 oz light cream cheese
3/4 cup granulated sugar
2 tbsp vegetable oil
2 tbsp margarine or butter
1 tsp vanilla
1 2/3 cups all-purpose flour
1/3 cup low-fat sour cream

Preheat the oven to 350°F. Spray two baking sheets with vegetable spray.

1. In a food processor, place cream cheese, sugar, oil, margarine, and vanilla. Purée until the mixture is smooth. Add flour and sour cream and pulse on and off until the mixture is crumbly. Remove it and form it into a ball. Wrap it with plastic wrap. Chill at least 20 minutes.
2. Between two sheets of floured waxed paper, roll the ball into a circle 1/8-inch thick. Using your favourite cookie cutters that are approximately 2 inches in diameter, cut out shapes and place them on prepared baking sheets. If you like, sprinkle with your favourite topping. Re-roll the scraps and repeat.
3. Bake for 15 to 18 minutes or until the cookies are light golden.

MAKES ABOUT
30 COOKIES

NUTRITIONAL ANALYSIS
PER COOKIE
Energy 58 calories
Protein 0.8 g
Fat, total 2.1 g
Fat, saturated 0.4 g
Carbohydrates 9 g
Fibre 0.1 g
Cholesterol 1.5 mg

NUTRITION WATCH
Traditional cut-out cookies are made primarily with butter or shortening and have lots of calories, cholesterol, and fat. My version comes in at about 75% fewer calories and less fat than the traditional cookies — the light cream cheese replaces some of that fat.

TIP
You can make this dough in advance and freeze it.

chocolate chip cookies

NUTRITIONAL ANALYSIS
PER COOKIE
Energy 80 calories
Protein 0.9 g
Fat, total 2.7 g
Fat, saturated 0.6 g
Carbohydrates 13 g
Fibre 0.3 g
Cholesterol 8.9 mg

NUTRITION WATCH
Regular chocolate chip cookies have three times the fat
and calories because of all
the butter or shortening,
eggs, and chocolate chips.

TIP
I often make this batter in
advance, freeze it, then bake
the cookies right out of the
freezer — a great quick, late-
night treat.

Chocolate chip cookies are an all-time favourite. I add extra vanilla to boost the flavour.
You'll never notice the fat is reduced.

1/3 cup granulated sugar
1/3 cup packed brown sugar
3 tbsp vegetable oil
1 large egg
2 tbsp corn syrup
1 tbsp vanilla
1 cup all-purpose flour
1/2 tsp baking powder
1/8 tsp salt
1/3 cup semi-sweet chocolate chips

Preheat the oven to 350°F. Spray two baking sheets with vegetable spray.

1. In a large bowl, combine sugar, brown sugar, oil, egg, corn syrup, and vanilla.
2. In another bowl, stir together flour, baking powder and salt. With a wooden spoon, stir the dry
    mixture into the wet ingredients until everything is combined. Stir in the chocolate chips.
3. Drop by the tbsp onto prepared baking sheets.
4. Bake for 12 to 15 minutes or until the cookies are golden.

peanut butter chip cookies

Peanut butter chips are sold in most grocery stores today. They make the difference in this cookie.

1/2 cup packed brown sugar
1/2 cup granulated sugar
1 large egg
1 tsp vanilla
1/3 cup smooth peanut butter
3 tbsp vegetable oil
1/4 cup low-fat milk
1 1/4 cups all-purpose flour
1/2 tsp baking powder
1/2 tsp baking soda
1/4 cup peanut butter chips

Preheat the oven to 350°F. Spray two baking sheets with vegetable spray.

1. In a large bowl and using a whisk or electric beater, mix brown sugar, sugar, egg, vanilla, peanut butter, oil, and milk.
2. In another bowl, stir together flour, baking powder, and baking soda. With a wooden spoon, stir the mixture into the wet ingredients just until everything is combined. Stir in the peanut butter chips.
3. Drop by the tbsp onto prepared baking sheets.
4. Bake for 12 to 15 minutes. Remove to a wire rack to cool.

MAKES ABOUT
36 COOKIES

NUTRITIONAL ANALYSIS
PER COOKIE
Energy 72 calories
Protein 1.5 g
Fat, total 2.9 g
Fat, saturated 0.5 g
Carbohydrates 10 g
Fibre 0.4 g
Cholesterol 6 mg

NUTRITION WATCH
Peanut butter, when combined with a grain such as bread, is a complete protein — wonderful for vegetarians.

TIPS
Be sure to buy natural peanut butter, not commercial, which is loaded with icing sugar and hydrogenated fat.

You can use regular chocolate chips instead of peanut butter chips in this recipe.

white chocolate chip cookies

These chocolate cookies have white chocolate chips spread throughout that melt into the cookies while they're baking. They're divinely delicious.

3/4 cup granulated sugar
1 large egg
3 tbsp vegetable oil
2 tbsp water
1 1/2 tbsp corn syrup
1 tsp vanilla
1 cup all-purpose flour
1/4 cup unsweetened cocoa powder
1/2 tsp baking powder
1/3 cup white chocolate chips

Preheat the oven to 350°F. Spray two baking sheets with vegetable spray.

1. In a large bowl and using a whisk or electric beater, combine sugar, egg, oil, water, corn syrup, and vanilla.
2. In another bowl, stir together flour, cocoa, and baking powder. With a wooden spoon, stir the mixture into the wet ingredients just until everything is combined. Stir in the chocolate chips.
3. Drop by the tbsp, spaced well apart, onto prepared baking sheets.
4. Bake one sheet at a time in the centre of the oven for 12 minutes or until the cookies are golden and slightly soft.

crisp chocolate oatmeal cookies

I find that adding corn syrup to the batter makes for a better-textured cookie. The oatmeal gives a crunchy texture.

1/2 cup packed brown sugar
1/4 cup granulated sugar
3 tbsp vegetable oil
2 tbsp corn syrup
1 large egg
1 tsp vanilla
3/4 cup quick-cooking oats
1/2 cup all-purpose flour
1/4 cup unsweetened cocoa powder
1/2 tsp baking soda

Preheat the oven to 350°F. Spray two baking sheets with vegetable spray.

1. In a large bowl and using a whisk or electric beater, combine brown sugar, sugar, oil, corn syrup, egg, and vanilla.
2. In another bowl, stir together oats, flour, cocoa, and baking soda. With a wooden spoon, stir the mixture into the wet ingredients until everything is combined.
3. Drop by the spoonful, about 2 inches apart, onto prepared baking sheets.
4. Bake for 12 minutes for a softer cookie, 15 minutes for a crisper cookie.

MAKES ABOUT
24 COOKIES

NUTRITIONAL ANALYSIS
PER COOKIE
Energy 72 calories
Protein 1.1 g
Fat, total 2.2 g
Fat, saturated 0.3 g
Carbohydrates 12 g
Fibre 0.6 g
Cholesterol 8.9 mg

NUTRITION WATCH
Oats are high in vitamin B1 and contain a good amount of vitamins B2 and E. Oatmeal is considered a low glycemic food, which causes your blood sugar to rise slowly, which in turn keeps you feeling full longer.

TIP
Use either quick-cooking rolled oats or old-fashioned oats in baking. Avoid instant oats, which can make the batter sticky.

crispy oatmeal lace cookies

These fine-textured cookies are fabulous right out of the oven. Use parchment paper because they tend to stick to the pan, even if it is well coated.

1/2 cup packed brown sugar
3 tbsp corn syrup
1 large egg
2 tbsp vegetable oil
1 tbsp margarine or butter
1 1/2 tsp vanilla
1 cup quick-cooking oats
3 tbsp all-purpose flour
1/2 tsp baking powder
1/8 tsp salt

Preheat the oven to 350°F. Line two baking sheets with parchment paper and spray with vegetable spray.

1. In a bowl and using a whisk or electric beater, combine brown sugar, corn syrup, egg, oil, margarine, and vanilla.
2. In another bowl, stir together oats, flour, baking powder, and salt. With a wooden spoon, stir the mixture into the wet ingredients until everything is combined.
3. Drop by the tbsp, 3 to 4 inches apart, onto prepared baking sheets.
4. Bake for 12 minutes or until the cookies are golden.

crunchy oatmeal dried cranberry cookies

The combination of oatmeal, Grape-Nuts cereal, and dried cranberries makes a wonderfully crisp and light cookie. I love it with my coffee in the morning.

3/4 cup packed brown sugar

3 tbsp vegetable oil

1 1/2 tbsp corn syrup

1 large egg

1 1/2 tsp vanilla

1/2 cup all-purpose flour

1/2 cup quick-cooking oats

1/2 cup Grape-Nuts cereal

1/2 cup dried cranberries

1 tsp baking powder

1/8 tsp salt

Preheat the oven to 350°F. Line two baking sheets with parchment paper and spray with vegetable spray.

1. In a large bowl and using a whisk or electric beater, combine brown sugar, oil, corn syrup, egg, and vanilla.
2. In another bowl, stir together flour, oats, cereal, cranberries, baking powder, and salt. With a wooden spoon, stir the mixture into the wet ingredients just until everything is combined.
3. Drop by the tbsp, spaced well apart, onto prepared baking sheets.
4. Bake in the centre of the oven for 10 to 12 minutes or until the cookies are golden and still slightly soft. Cool them on the baking sheet for several minutes before transferring them to a wire rack.

MAKES ABOUT
24 COOKIES

NUTRITIONAL ANALYSIS
PER COOKIE
Energy 83 calories
Protein 1 g
Fat, total 2.1 g
Fat, saturated 0.2 g
Carbohydrates 15 g
Fibre 0.7 g
Cholesterol 8.9 mg

NUTRITION WATCH
Grape-Nuts cereal is a tasty low-fat breakfast cereal made from wheat and toasted barley. It's ideal to use in baking because it adds a nut-like texture without the fat and calories of nuts.

TIP
Use any dried fruit you like. Diced apricots, dates, or prunes go well with these cookies.

peanut butter and jam cookies

Who needs peanut butter and jam sandwiches when you can have these delicious cookies? The spiral look make these so attractive.

3/4 cup packed brown sugar
1/4 cup smooth peanut butter
3 tbsp corn syrup
2 tbsp vegetable oil
1 large egg
1 tsp vanilla
1 1/3 cups all-purpose flour
2 tbsp cornstarch
3/4 tsp baking powder
1/4 cup raspberry jam

Preheat the oven to 350°F. Spray two baking sheets with vegetable spray.

1. In a large bowl and using a whisk or electric beater, combine brown sugar, peanut butter, corn syrup, oil, egg, and vanilla.
2. In another bowl, stir together flour, cornstarch, and baking powder. With a wooden spoon, stir the mixture into the peanut butter mixture just until everything is combined. Divide the dough into two balls and wrap them in plastic wrap. Chill for 20 minutes.
3. Between two sheets of floured waxed paper, roll one ball of dough into a rectangle 1/8-inch thick. Repeat with the other ball.
4. Remove the top pieces of waxed paper. Spread the jam evenly over both rectangles. Starting from the long end and using waxed paper to assist, roll each rectangle up tightly, jelly roll–fashion. Slice into 1/2-inch slices. Place the cut side down on prepared baking sheets.
5. Bake in the centre of the oven for 18 to 20 minutes or until the cookies are lightly browned.

MAKES ABOUT
24 COOKIES

NUTRITIONAL ANALYSIS
PER COOKIE
Energy 99 calories
Protein 1.6 g
Fat, total 2.7 g
Fat, saturated 0.3 g
Carbohydrates 17 g
Fibre 0.4 g
Cholesterol 8.9 mg

NUTRITION WATCH
Peanut butter is a highly nutritious snack for children and adults. Even though it contains 100 calories and 8 g of fat per tbsp, it is considered a healthy (monounsaturated) fat. Eat it in moderation.

TIP
Chilling the dough makes it easier to roll. But if you're in a hurry, drop the dough by the spoonful on a baking sheet, put a small amount of jam in the middle of each cookie, and bake 12 minutes or just until the cookies are lightly browned.

marble wafers

These cookies are beautiful to serve and delicious to eat. The two-tone look makes them appealing to kids as well.

1/4 cup vegetable oil

2 tbsp corn syrup

1 large egg

2 tsp vanilla

3/4 cup granulated sugar

1/8 tsp salt

1/2 tsp baking powder

1 cup all-purpose flour

2 tbsp granulated sugar

2 tbsp unsweetened cocoa powder

Preheat the oven to 350°F. Spray two baking sheets with vegetable spray.

1. In a large bowl and using a whisk or electric beater, combine oil, corn syrup, egg, vanilla, 3/4 cup sugar, and salt. Divide the mixture in half.
2. To one half, add 1/4 tsp of the baking powder and 2/3 cup of the flour; with a wooden spoon, stir until everything is combined.
3. To the other half, add 2 tbsp sugar; stir until everything is combined. Stir in cocoa, remaining baking powder, and remaining flour until combined.
4. Take 1 tsp of each of the dark and light doughs; press them together and place them on prepared baking sheets. Repeat with remaining dough.
5. Bake in the centre of the oven for 10 to 12 minutes or until the cookies are lightly browned.

MAKES ABOUT
30 COOKIES

NUTRITIONAL ANALYSIS
PER COOKIE
Energy 62 calories
Protein 0.7 g
Fat, total 2.1 g
Fat, saturated 0.2 g
Carbohydrates 10 g
Fibre 0.2 g
Cholesterol 7.1 mg

NUTRITION WATCH
In most cookie recipes, the primary ingredient is fat, either from butter, oil, or vegetable shortening. Most traditional recipes contain as much as 1 cup of fat. One tablespoon of fat contains approximately 120 calories and 14 g of fat. I reduce the fat in my cookies by at least 50%.

TIP
Corn syrup gives this cookie a softer texture. Low-fat cookies at times can be dry or too crisp.

ginger snaps

The flavouring of a gingerbread cookie is such a traditional one, with the most common ingredient being molasses and cinnamon. These ginger snaps are simple yet addictive.

3/4 cup packed brown sugar
1/2 tsp ground cinnamon
1/4 tsp ground ginger
2 tbsp margarine or butter
2 tbsp vegetable oil
2 tbsp molasses
1 large egg
1 cup all-purpose flour
1/2 tsp baking soda

Preheat the oven to 350°F. Spray two baking sheets with vegetable spray.

1. In a large bowl and using a whisk or electric beater, combine brown sugar, cinnamon, ginger, margarine, oil, molasses, and egg.
2. In another bowl, stir together flour and baking soda. With a wooden spoon, stir the mixture into the wet ingredients until everything is combined.
3. Drop by the tbsp, spaced well apart, onto prepared baking sheets.
4. Bake one sheet at a time in the centre of the oven for 10 to 12 minutes or until the cookies are golden brown and still slightly soft.

MAKES ABOUT
30 COOKIES

NUTRITIONAL ANALYSIS
PER COOKIE
Energy 58 calories
Protein 0.7 g
Fat, total 1.9 g
Fat, saturated 0.3 g
Carbohydrates 9.5 g
Fibre 0.1 g
Cholesterol 7.1 mg

NUTRITION WATCH
You can substitute 2 egg whites for the whole egg, if you want to reduce the fat and cholesterol from the yolk.

TIP
For spicier cookies, add a dash of nutmeg, allspice, and cloves.

molasses mocha crisps

Molasses and coffee make a divine combination, especially in a cookie.

2 tsp instant coffee granules
1/4 cup hot water
3 tbsp corn syrup
2 tbsp vegetable oil
2 tbsp molasses
1 tbsp margarine or butter
1/2 cup packed brown sugar
3/4 cup all-purpose flour
1/4 tsp ground cinnamon
1/4 tsp ground ginger

Preheat the oven to 350°F. Spray two baking sheets with vegetable spray.

1. Dissolve the instant coffee in hot water. In a large bowl and using a whisk or electric beaters, combine coffee, corn syrup, oil, molasses, butter, and brown sugar.
2. In another bowl, stir together flour, cinnamon, and ginger. With a wooden spoon, stir the mixture into the wet ingredients until everything is combined.
3. Drop by the spoonful, spaced 3 inches apart, onto prepared baking sheets.
4. Bake one sheet at a time for 10 to 12 minutes or until the cookies are golden and slightly soft.

MAKES ABOUT
24 COOKIES

NUTRITIONAL ANALYSIS
PER COOKIE
Energy 61 calories
Protein 0.4 g
Fat, total 1.7 g
Fat, saturated 0.2 g
Carbohydrates 11 g
Fibre 0.1 g
Cholesterol 0

NUTRITION WATCH
Molasses contains iron, calcium, and phosphorous.

TIP
You can substitute the instant coffee with strong brewed left over from breakfast.

lemon poppyseed crisps

These lemon cookies are crisp and bursting with flavour. The addition of corn syrup gives the cookies a better texture, so the excess fat is not missed.

MAKES ABOUT
22 COOKIES

NUTRITIONAL ANALYSIS
PER COOKIE
Energy 90 calories
Protein 1.2 g
Fat, total 2.4 g
Fat, saturated 0.3 g
Carbohydrates 16 g
Fibre 0.5 g
Cholesterol 9.7 mg

NUTRITION WATCH
Lemons are an excellent
source of vitamin C. Use soon
after squeezing, or their
vitamin power is reduced.

TIP
For any recipe depending
upon lemon for the number-
one flavour, as in this cookie,
always use freshly squeezed
juice. The bottled version is
inferior.

1 cup granulated sugar
3 tbsp vegetable oil
1 tbsp finely grated lemon rind
3 tbsp fresh lemon juice
2 tbsp corn syrup
1 large egg
1 tsp vanilla
2/3 cup all-purpose flour
3/4 cup quick-cooking oats
1 tsp poppyseeds
1 tsp baking powder
1/8 tsp salt

Preheat the oven to 350°F. Spray two baking sheets with vegetable spray.

1. In a bowl and using a whisk or electric beater, combine sugar, oil, lemon rind and juice, corn syrup, egg, and vanilla.
2. In another bowl, stir together flour, oats, poppyseeds, baking powder, and salt. With a wooden spoon, stir the mixture into the wet ingredients until everything is combined.
3. Drop by the tbsp, about 3 inches apart, onto prepared baking sheets.
4. Bake for 12 minutes or until the cookies are lightly browned.

white chocolate chip biscotti

In my other cookbooks, I always include one or two biscotti recipes. I'm so thrilled that I can play with so many different flavours! The white chips melt into this cookie.

3/4 cup granulated sugar
1/4 cup margarine or butter, softened
1 large egg
2 large egg whites
2 tbsp chocolate syrup
1 tsp vanilla
1 3/4 cups all-purpose flour
1/4 cup unsweetened cocoa powder
1/3 cup white chocolate chips
2 tsp baking powder

Preheat the oven to 350°F. Spray two baking sheets with vegetable spray.

1. In a food processor or bowl, combine sugar, margarine, egg, egg whites, chocolate syrup, and vanilla; process until the mixture is smooth.
2. With a wooden spoon, stir in flour, cocoa, chocolate chips, and baking powder just until everything is combined. Divide the dough in half. Shape each half into a log 12 x 4 inches. Place the logs well apart on a baking sheet.
3. Bake for 20 minutes. Remove the sheet from the oven. Let the logs cool on the sheet for 5 minutes.
4. Transfer the logs to a cutting board. Slice them on the diagonal into 1/2-inch-thick cookies. Place the cookies flat on prepared baking sheets. Bake them for 15 minutes longer.

MAKES ABOUT
30 COOKIES

NUTRITIONAL ANALYSIS
PER COOKIE
Energy 61 calories
Protein 1.1 g
Fat, total 1.9 g
Fat, saturated 0.6 g
Carbohydrates 9.8 g
Fibre 0.4 g
Cholesterol 5.6 mg

NUTRITION WATCH
By using egg whites, you eliminate the fat and cholesterol from the yolk. In most recipes, I like to use one whole egg and substitute any other whole egg with two egg whites to reduce the fat and cholesterol.

TIP
Chocolate syrup gives these cookies more chocolate flavour without added fat or cholesterol. You can use store-bought syrup or make the Chocolate Sauce on page 240.

orange pecan biscotti

To get the most intense orange flavour, I use orange juice concentrate, rather than orange juice. Keep a can in the freezer at all times, just for baking and cooking.

1 1/4 cup granulated sugar
2 large eggs
1/4 cup vegetable oil
5 tbsp orange juice concentrate
2 tsp finely grated orange rind
1 1/2 tsp vanilla
2 cups all-purpose flour
1 1/2 tsp baking powder
1/8 tsp salt
1/3 cup chopped toasted pecans

Preheat the oven to 350°F. Spray a baking sheet with vegetable spray.

1. In a large bowl and with a whisk or electric beater, combine sugar, eggs, oil, orange juice concentrate, orange rind, and vanilla.
2. With a wooden spoon, stir in flour, baking powder, salt, and pecans just until everything is combined. Divide the dough in half. Shape each half into a 12-inch × 4-inch log. Place the logs well apart on a baking sheet.
3. Bake for 20 minutes. Remove the sheet from the oven and let the logs cool on the sheet for 5 minutes.
4. Transfer the logs to a cutting board. Slice them on the diagonal into 1/2-inch thick cookies. Place the cookies flat on the baking sheet. Bake for 15 minutes longer or until they are crisp and lightly browned.

mocha chip biscotti

Coffee and chocolate go so well together. I enjoy these cookies as a late-morning snack, with a low-fat caffé latte.

2 tsp instant coffee granules
1/4 cup hot water
2/3 cup packed brown sugar
1/4 cup granulated sugar
1/3 cup vegetable oil
2 large eggs
2 tsp vanilla
2 1/3 cups all-purpose flour
1/3 cup semi-sweet chocolate chips
2 tsp baking powder

Preheat the oven to 350°F. Spray a baking sheet with vegetable spray.

1. Dissolve the instant coffee in the hot water.
2. In a bowl and using a whisk or electric beater, combine coffee, brown sugar, sugar, oil, eggs, and vanilla.
3. With a wooden spoon, stir in flour, chocolate chips, and baking powder just until everything is combined. Divide the dough in half. Shape each half into a 12-inch × 4-inch log. Place the logs well apart on a baking sheet.
4. Bake for 20 minutes. Remove the sheet from the oven and let cool for 5 minutes.
5. Transfer the logs to a cutting board. Slice them on the diagonal into 1/2-inch thick cookies. Place the cookies flat on the baking sheet. Bake for 15 minutes longer.

MAKES ABOUT
36 COOKIES

NUTRITIONAL ANALYSIS
PER COOKIE
Energy 76 calories
Protein 1.3 g
Fat, total 2.8 g
Fat, saturated 0.5 g
Carbohydrates 12 g
Fibre 0.4 g
Cholesterol 11.7 mg

NUTRITION WATCH
The stronger the coffee, the less caffeine, so the occasional espresso is better for you than regular coffee.

TIP
If you have some left-over brewed coffee from breakfast, use 1/4 cup instead of instant coffee.

mint fudge meringues

MAKES ABOUT
20 COOKIES

NUTRITIONAL ANALYSIS
PER COOKIE
Energy 30 calories
Protein 0.4 g
Fat, total 0.4 g
Fat, saturated 0.3 g
Carbohydrates 6.1 g
Fibre 0.3 g
Cholesterol 0

NUTRITION WATCH
Meringues are the lowest fat
cookies you can enjoy. There's
never any oil or butter them.

TIP
Don't overuse mint extract
because it has a powerful
intensity — 1/4 tsp is all you
need.

Another heavenly variation of a meringue cookie. The mint flavour is subtle and delicious.

2 large egg whites
1/4 tsp cream of tartar
1/2 cup granulated sugar
2 tbsp unsweetened cocoa powder
1 1/2 tsp cornstarch
1/4 tsp mint extract
2 tbsp semi-sweet mint chocolate chips

Preheat the oven to 275°F. Line a baking sheet with parchment paper.

1. In a bowl and using a whisk or electric beater, beat the egg whites until they are foamy. Add the cream of tartar and beat until soft peaks form. Gradually add sugar, continuing to beat until stiff peaks form.
2. Beat in cocoa, cornstarch, and mint extract. Fold in the mint chocolate chips.
3. Drop by the tbsp onto a prepared baking sheet. Bake 1 hour or until the meringues are dry.

sauces

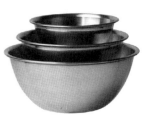

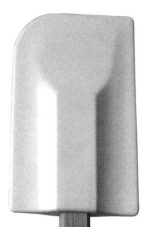

tips for divine light sauces

1. Dessert sauces are a very individual choice. If you like an accompaniment to your dessert, select one that matches well. For example, strawberry or raspberry sauce always goes well with chocolate desserts or fruit-based desserts. Chocolate sauce goes well with chocolate, lemon, orange or berry desserts.

2. When you're working with cornstarch, always add it to a cold base and mix until it is incorporated and the sauce is smooth. Then heat it on medium until it is slightly thickened. Be careful not to burn the sauce.

3. When you add an egg to a sauce, always pour the hot sauce into the whisked egg and pour the mixture back into the saucepan, keeping it on a low heat and whisking constantly until the mixture is thickened. If not, you'll cook the egg. If the egg cooks or curdles, the heat was too high, and you'll have to start again.

4. When you're cooling a sauce, place some plastic wrap over top to prevent a skin from forming.

5. Cooked sauces usually thicken upon cooling. If you want a looser consistency, heat it gently in the microwave, for approximately 20 to 30 seconds. You can also add a little milk or other liquid to the recipe.

caramel sauce

This is a great sauce to serve over any dessert featuring apples or chocolate.

1/2 cup packed brown sugar
1/4 cup skim evaporated milk
1 1/2 tbsp corn syrup
2 tsp margarine or butter

1. In a small saucepan, whisk together brown sugar, evaporated milk, corn syrup, and margarine. Cook over the lowest heat for 5 minutes, stirring constantly, or until the sauce is smooth and slightly thickened.
2. Pour the sauce into a bowl. Cover and chill.

MAKES ABOUT 3/4 CUP

NUTRITIONAL ANALYSIS
PER TBSP
Energy 52 calories
Protein 0.4 g
Fat, total 0.7 g
Fat, saturated 0.4 g
Carbohydrates 11 g
Fibre 0
Cholesterol 1.9 mg

crème anglaise

This light and creamy sauce is wonderful over bread puddings and pudding cakes. In fact, I serve it over any dessert that tastes best when it comes right out of the oven, such as phyllo desserts, soufflés, crisps, and cobblers.

1/3 cup granulated sugar
1 large egg
1 tsp vanilla
3/4 cup 2% milk

1. In a bowl, whisk together sugar, egg, and vanilla.
2. In a small saucepan, heat the milk over medium heat until it is steaming. Gradually add it to the egg mixture, whisking constantly. Return the mixture to the saucepan. Cook over low heat, stirring constantly, for 5 to 8 minutes or until it is slightly thickened. Do not boil.
3. Pour the sauce into a bowl. Place a piece of plastic wrap on the surface of the sauce. Chill.

MAKES ABOUT 1 CUP

NUTRITIONAL ANALYSIS
PER TBSP
Energy 27 calories
Protein 0.8 g
Fat, total 0.5 g
Fat, saturated 0.2 g
Carbohydrates 48 g
Fibre 0
Cholesterol 14 mg

chocolate sauce

This is my basic low-fat chocolate sauce, which I love over almost any dessert. It goes well with other chocolate- and fruit-based desserts, as well as with cheesecakes, soufflés, jelly rolls, coffee cakes … just about any dessert!

1/3 cup granulated sugar
3 tbsp unsweetened cocoa powder
1/4 cup corn syrup
1/4 cup water

1. In a small saucepan, whisk together sugar, cocoa, corn syrup, and water. Bring the mixture to a boil. Reduce the heat and simmer for 5 minutes or until it is slightly thickened.
2. Pour the sauce into a bowl and cover.

dark chocolate orange sauce

This is a variation of my basic chocolate sauce with the addition of orange juice concentrate and orange zest, which contribute an intense orange flavour.

1/3 cup granulated sugar
3 tbsp unsweetened cocoa powder
1/4 cup corn syrup
1/4 cup water
2 tbsp orange juice concentrate
2 tsp finely grated orange rind

1. In a small saucepan, whisk together sugar, cocoa, corn syrup, water, orange juice concentrate, and orange rind. Bring the mixture to a boil, stirring. Reduce the heat to low; simmer for 5 minutes or until the sauce is slightly thickened.
2. Pour it into a bowl and cover.

chocolate raspberry sauce

This is another variation of my basic chocolate sauce. The addition of raspberry jam gives this sauce a great flavour and texture.

1/3 cup granulated sugar
3 tbsp unsweetened cocoa powder
1/4 cup corn syrup
1/4 cup water
3 tbsp raspberry jam

1. In a small saucepan, whisk together sugar, cocoa, corn syrup, water, and jam. Bring the mixture to a boil. Reduce the heat and simmer for 3 minutes or until the sauce is slightly thickened.
2. Pour the sauce into a bowl and cover.

MAKES ABOUT 1 CUP

NUTRITIONAL ANALYSIS
PER TBSP
Energy 46 calories
Protein 0.2 g
Fat, total 0.1 g
Fat, saturated 0.1 g
Carbohydrates 11 g
Fibre 0.3 g
Cholesterol 0

vanilla cream

This light, creamy sauce tastes fabulous over many of the pies and tart recipes in this book. It tastes like a light Devon cream.

2 tbsp granulated sugar
1/2 cup low-fat vanilla yogurt
1 oz light cream cheese, softened
1/2 tsp vanilla

1. In a food processor, combine sugar, yogurt, cream cheese, and vanilla; purée until the mixture is smooth.
2. Pour the sauce into a bowl. Cover and chill.

MAKES ABOUT 3/4 CUP

NUTRITIONAL ANALYSIS
PER TBSP
Energy 23 calories
Protein 0.8 g
Fat, total 0.5 g
Fat, saturated 0.3 g
Carbohydrates 3.7 g
Fibre 0
Cholesterol 1.8 mg

strawberry coulis

A coulis is a general term referring to a thick purée or sauce. This strawberry sauce is heavenly on any chocolate or fruit-based dessert.

8 oz fresh or frozen strawberries
1/4 cup icing sugar
2 tbsp water

1. If using frozen berries, thaw and drain them well.
2. In a food processor, combine berries, icing sugar, and water; purée until the mixture is smooth.

MAKES ABOUT 1 CUP

NUTRITIONAL ANALYSIS
PER TBSP

Energy 13 calories

Protein 0.1 g

Fat, total 0.1 g

Fat, saturated 0

Carbohydrates 2.9 g

Fibre 0.3 g

Cholesterol 0

raspberry coulis

This thick and rich-tasting sauce is wonderful over any chocolate dessert, soufflé, or fruit-based dessert.

8 oz fresh or frozen raspberries
1/3 cup icing sugar
2 tbsp water

1. If using frozen berries, thaw and drain them well.
2. In a food processor, combine berries, icing sugar, and water; purée until the mixture is smooth.

MAKES ABOUT 1 CUP

NUTRITIONAL ANALYSIS
PER TBSP

Energy 18 calories

Protein 0.1 g

Fat, total 0.1 g

Fat, saturated 0

Carbohydrates 4.1 g

Fibre 0.4 g

Cholesterol 0

mango coulis

A mango sauce goes well over any fruit-based dessert, such as those with apricots or berries. It's also wonderful with any chocolate dessert.

1 ripe mango, peeled, pitted, and diced
3 tbsp icing sugar
2 tbsp orange juice

1. In a food processor, combine mango, icing sugar, and orange juice; purée until the mixture is smooth.
2. Pour the sauce into a bowl. Cover and chill.

MAKES ABOUT 1 CUP

NUTRITIONAL ANALYSIS
PER TBSP
Energy 16 calories
Protein 0.1 g
Fat, total 0
Fat, saturated 0
Carbohydrates 3.8 g
Fibre 0.2 g
Cholesterol 0

lemon sauce

This citrus sauce is heavenly with chocolate desserts or lemon soufflés.

1/2 cup granulated sugar
1 1/2 tbsp cornstarch
2/3 cup orange juice
1 tsp finely grated lemon rind
3 tbsp fresh lemon juice

1. In a small saucepan off the heat, whisk together sugar, cornstarch, orange juice, lemon rind, and lemon juice until the mixture is smooth. Bring it to a boil. Reduce the heat and simmer for 4 minutes or until the sauce is thickened.
2. Pour the sauce into a bowl and cover.

MAKES ABOUT 3/4 CUP

NUTRITIONAL ANALYSIS
PER TBSP
Energy 44 calories
Protein 0.1 g
Fat, total 0
Fat, saturated 0
Carbohydrates 11 g
Fibre 0.1 g
Cholesterol 0

fruit glaze

MAKES ABOUT 3 TBSP

NUTRITIONAL ANALYSIS
PER SERVING
(OF 8-SLICE CAKE)
Energy 14 calories
Protein 0
Fat, total 0
Fat, saturated 0
Carbohydrates 3.5 g
Fibre 0
Cholesterol 0

A fruit-decorated dessert always looks best if it is glazed before serving.

2 tbsp apple jelly or red currant jelly
1 tbsp water

1. In small microwavable bowl, combine jelly and water. Microwave on high for 30 seconds. Stir until the mixture is smooth.
2. Brush over berries or sliced fruit on top of a cheesecake or tart.

ready-to-serve sauce

MAKES 1 CUP

NUTRITIONAL ANALYSIS
PER TBSP
Energy 15 calories
Protein 0.6 g
Fat, total 0.2 g
Fat, saturated 0.2 g
Carbohydrates 0.2 g
Fibre 0.2 g
Cholesterol 0.6 mg

This is the easiest sauce you can make. I often keep containers of frozen yogurt, ice, or sorbet on hand, usually chocolate, raspberry, lemon, and mango.

1 cup low-fat chocolate frozen yogurt or other frozen yogurt or sherbet of your choice

1. Place the frozen yogurt in bowl. Let it stand until it has melted, stirring occasionally.

index

rhubarb strawberry granola crisp, 81
rice puddings
  chocolate, 163
  with dates and apricots, 164
ricotta cheese, as ingredient, 14–15
rind, 16
rolls
  apricot, 168
  banana, with chocolate filling, 182
  jelly. *See* jelly rolls
  mocha, 169
rugelach
  apricot jam cranberry, 219
  chocolate, 220
rum raisin coconut pudding, 117

S

salt, 5
sauces
  caramel, 239
  chocolate, 240
  chocolate raspberry, 241
  crème anglaise, 239
  dark chocolate orange, 240
  fruit glaze, 244
  lemon, 243
  mango coulis, 243
  raspberry coulis, 242
  ready-to-serve, 244
  strawberry coulis, 242
  tips, 238

vanilla cream, 241
scones
  apricot orange, 215
  blueberry sour cream, 214
  tips, 204
shortbread
  cheesecake squares, 131
  pecan tarts, 104
soufflés
  chocolate, 107
  lemon, 110
  mocha Irish cream, 109
  orange, 108
  tips, 106
sour cream
  apple pie, 159
  blueberry peach cobbler, 80
  blueberry scones, 214
  brownie cheesecake, 45
  chocolate cake, 30
  chocolate cheesecake squares, 132
  cranberry coffee cake, 53
  as ingredient, 14
  orange apple coffee cake, 54
soy desserts
  apple cinnamon noodle pudding
    cake, 165
  apricot roll, 168
  banana chocolate meringue pie, 158
  banana marble coffee cake, 156
  Irish cream chocolate pudding, 161
  lemon cheesecake, 155
  lemon poppyseed loaf, 170

strawberry, glazed, 42

streusel, 65

turnovers, date, 192

U

upside-down cakes

apple and cranberry, 57

orange, 66

utensils, 19

V

vanilla cream, 241

vegetable oil spray, 9

vegetable oils, 9

W

wafers, marble, 229

walnut and maple syrup pudding, 120

Y

yogurt, 13

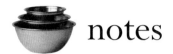

notes

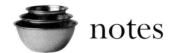

notes

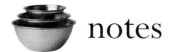

notes

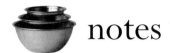 notes